The
Natural Medicine
Guidebook

How to Source, Grow, and Make Your Own Herbal Remedies, Including Teas, Essential Oils, and Infusions

Stephen H. Sharp

Table of Contents

Medical disclaimer: This book is not meant to replace medical treatment.

Introduction

When we hear the term "Big Pharma," it is so easy to underestimate the actual monetary value of the pharmaceutical industry. The reality is that most people know that every time they are filling a prescription, they are settling for an option that is likely overpriced and is increasing the wealth of those at the helm of this multimillion dollar industry. Yet, as the value of the pharmaceutical industry is so immense, the true value of the industry can be hard to fathom for the ordinary man and woman in the street. So, what are the true values I am referring to here? Statistics indicate that the pharmaceutical market in the US alone is valued at $575.5 billion. This number sets the US far ahead of any other country, as in second position, we have China at $118.8 billion (Mikulic, 2023).

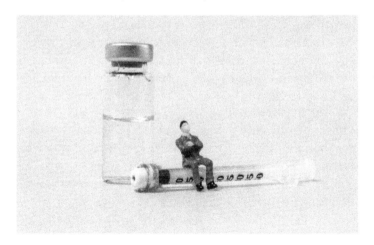

Does it feel like there is very little you can do about this immense wealth generation and large companies profiteering from the needs of the ordinary citizen? Yes, for most people, it does feel that way, and understandably so. However, there is something you do have control over. You may not be able to change the world and the ways in which this industry operates, but you can minimize the financial impact it has on your budget by opting out of supporting this trade. You have the freedom to choose whether you want to contribute your hard-earned cash to this wealth generation, or whether you would rather turn your focus to gaining greater familiarity with natural remedies and increasing confidence in using this much more affordable alternative. You also have control over the choice to ignore the warnings of possible side effects listed in fine print on lengthy pamphlets that are folded tightly inside the packaging of the prescription you are taking home, or to opt for the natural route—a route that, in most cases, isn't threatening to cause as much harm as good.

For those who are keen to settle for the latter options, the greatest obstacle they have to overcome is a lack of knowledge about what natural remedies to use, how to use them, and how to gain optimal results from what is available to them.

These are the needs I have often come across during my journey as a health, fitness, nutrition, and medicine enthusiast. Even though these have been topics that piqued my interest for most of my life, it was roughly 14 years ago when I decided to shift my focus to my passion, and I actively started to study these health-related topics. It is how I increased my existing knowledge of natural medicine and how to source and make these remedies.

I am completely intrigued by the wonders you can find in natural remedies. The knowledge that we can find in nature is all we need to resolve many ailments and also improve our overall well-being. Nature's solution to medicine is by far more affordable than alternatives you'll find under the umbrella term of "modern medicine." Even better though is that natural medicine doesn't pose the same risks through the numerous side effects you'll commonly find in most prescriptions.

As a passionate enthusiast and an advocate for natural solutions to health and wellness, I share my knowledge, the cumulation of years of research, and the practical application of what I've learned in my life with you. We'll be covering the topic of natural medicine from several perspectives, starting this journey at its origin and comparing it with modern medicine. Then, in the second part of the book, I shift my approach to be more practical and, there, I'll be sharing guidelines on how to put together an apothecary at home and where and how to source your herbs. I am offering a guide on how to get started by growing your herbs, as well as the best methods when it comes to drying and storing them. I included an entire chapter on herbal remedies you can use for addressing many common ailments and specific herbal remedies you can use to ensure optimal mental and physical health. You'll even learn how to make tinctures and essential oils at home.

Lastly, I am covering tea as a form of herbal remedy through my teachings on how to prepare and store teas and what teas you need to take to improve various specific concerns.

If you are an enthusiast of natural medicine and would love to steer away from supporting Big Pharma, this book offers you a comprehensive collection of knowledge to get you going on this journey, and you'll be able to jump all in on this new journey. However, even if you are merely willing to dip your toe into the pool of possibilities, you'll find this book insightful too, as there are many solutions you can opt for. It will enable you to first gain greater confidence in the effectiveness of natural medicine before jumping all in.

This book is a work that resulted from my passion for natural remedies and choosing an alternative way to enjoy health and wellness in all areas of my life. I hope that my passion further ignites your flame to explore the possibilities available to you.

So, let's start at the beginning and step back in time to explore the origins of natural medicine.

Chapter 1:

Origins of Herbal Medicine

Throughout the history of humankind, there are several practices that societies relied on for mental and physical wellness. However, as time went by, these practices were often first supplemented with alternative approaches to healing until the latter eventually completely overshadowed the ancient practices, becoming completely marginalized. Yet, over more recent decades, there has been a revival, and interest in these aged practices is increasing globally. Herbal medicine is one such practice that was nearly forgotten until it became a point of interest in modern society again.

The History of Herbal Medicine

It is hard to pinpoint the exact era when people started to use herbs to treat various ailments, but historic records found in China show that we can say with relative certainty that it dates back to at least as far back as 2800 B.C.E. (Sturluson, 2014).

Since then, historians can pinpoint several eras showing records of herbs being used in this way across the globe, indicating a worldwide interest in the use of herbs for medicinal reasons.

In 400 B.C.E., it was the Greeks who had an herbal medicine game and Hippocrates who enlightened the nation to the benefits linked to healthy eating, exercise, and being in an overall state of joy, the pillars to lasting wellness. Cultivating herbs for medicinal purposes became the norm across the Roman Empire around the year 50 C.E., but it was only around the 200s that civilizations started to classify ailments and prescribed the use of specific herbal remedies to address certain diseases or medical concerns (Sturluson, 2014).

Next, we have to take a jump in the timeline over several centuries right into the monasteries where monks used herbal remedies to treat the sick, which was roughly around the year 800 C.E. We have the stories told in Homer's *The Iliad* and *The Odyssey*, describing plant species that can heal various diseases, and 300 years later, herbal medicine was mentioned in the *Canon of Medicine*, a work of the Arab doctor Avicenna. Not too long after this, the black death spread across the European continent in 1200, and several alternative remedies were mentioned as possible treatment options to this deadly disease (Sturluson, 2014).

From here onwards, the recordkeeping became more consistent and taught us that Henry VII was a keen supporter of herbalists; he and his parliament were keen to improve the standard of local apothecaries to ensure they provided better care. This took place around 1500, but only a mere 100 years later, herbal remedies were no longer the sought-after solution as there was no treatment option limited to caring for the poor, while the wealthy would opt for more expensive drugs (Sturluson, 2014).

The ideas that food should be our medicine and that it is possible to ensure holistic health and wellness by opting for healthy food choices have been around for quite some time. It was the message that Preacher Charles shared with the nation in the 1700s (Sturluson, 2014).

A century later, pharmaceuticals came onto the scene in a big way and cast a shadow over herbal remedies. Yet, even at this early age, there are already records documenting the side effects you may endure from opting for this more advanced form of treatment. The 1800s also marked the foundation of the National Association of Medicinal Herbalists, later known as the National Institute of Medical Herbalists (NIMH).

While it may appear as if herbal remedies were now almost pushed entirely onto the back burner, the need for supplies during WWI forced people to turn to herbs once again to treat the sick and injured. Soon after the war ended, pharmaceuticals became more available again, and this era marks the time when penicillin was discovered.

By the 1950s, the number of concerns over the impact that pharmaceuticals have in the form of side effects accumulated and turned into an uproar, resulting in having herbal practitioners reinstated along with the approval that was previously taken away.

Now, we are in the 2000s, and Big Pharma has a place in almost every home across the globe. One thing that remains a constant though is that the concern over side effects and the impact that pharmaceuticals have on the body remain pressing matters for many, and the number of concerned citizens is growing. Thus, over decades later, there is an uprise in the interest in finding effective herbal remedies to treat concerns, which ordinary people like you and me don't feel comfortable trusting pharmaceuticals with any longer.

By taking an overview of this timeline, it becomes evident that since the time that pharmaceuticals entered the scene, there has been a kind of coexisting relationship between natural medicine and the more modern alternative. This is a relationship where modern medicine has predominantly been dominating the scene, and the conventional perspective on medicine in its entirety seemed to consider herbal remedies as the inferior player in the field. Yet, just because it is the popular belief, it doesn't make it true. Throughout this book, you, too, will come to realize the immense healing abilities natural options have to offer.

Making this statement is not merely my opinion but a trend we can witness in official statistics too. It is the valuable contribution herbal medicine has to offer that has fueled its sharp increase in interest over the past couple of decades, especially in developed countries. It is also important to note that even though the use of herbs in their natural form may still be overshadowed by pharmaceuticals to an immense degree, certain active compounds of herbs are often used during the manufacturing processes of modern medicine (IARC Working Group on the Evaluation of Carcinogenic Risks to Humans, n.d.).

The Role of Herbal Medicine in Various Cultures

One thing we can say with absolute certainty is that the development of herbal medicine can't be linked to one single civilization. We can revert to ancient records indicating the role herbal medicine played in the history of cultures and societies from every populated continent in the world. As we delve deeper into how various cultures developed and used herbal remedies, it quickly becomes evident that the most popular approach was to use herbs as holistic medicine. Herbs and remedies derived from various plant parts played a contributing role in treating concerns linked to the mind, body, and soul. We also learn that the use of herbal medicine is not only linked to treating disease but also acting as a preventative measure to ensure optimal wellness, which is very similar to the way we still use it today.

The Americas

The history of herbal medicine is woven into the existence of the Native Americans. While the application methods varied from one tribe to another, it was mostly the case that herbal treatments were mostly part of a much larger process that included ceremonies and rituals. These tribes would consider physical ailments as concerns linked to the mental and spiritual state of the sick. They believed that health is only possible when the person is in a state of harmony. Thus, the use of herbal remedies was not only limited to treating wounds and physical diseases but also to curing concerns on a spiritual level. Studying herbs forms a large part of this culture and the result is that over thousands of years, Native Americans developed an immense wealth of knowledge of more than 500 plant species. Some of the herbs that were often used in their healing rituals are mint, magnolia, and milkweed (Adelmann, 2013).

India

When we look at cultures that have been contributing largely to the development of alternative medicine, we need to shift our focus to India, the place where Ayurvedic medicine originated. This is a medicinal practice dating back roughly 3,000 years. The term *Ayurveda* is derived from the Sanskrit words *ayur*, meaning "life," and *veda*, referring to "knowledge" or "science." The type of medicine has its roots in the Hindu tradition, and, when you explore the records dating back to this time, you'll learn that this type of medicine included several treatment types to address a wide range of concerns. It is a medicinal practice that is closely linked to religious rituals too. Ayurvedic medicine became so widely acclaimed that it even found a place in Western medicine.

Similar to the traditional healing we've explored with Native Americans, Ayurvedic medicine also consists of a holistic approach and includes meditation, massage, yoga, healthy eating, the use of essential oils, and even enemas along with herbal medicine. The method relies on the inclusion of minerals and metal substances along with herbal compounds. It is an alternative form of treatment that became quite advanced, and, within the framework of Ayurvedic medicine, we find that it included surgery, namely the extraction of kidney stones and rhinoplasty.

China

The Chinese medicinal practices can bring about a range of ethical concerns, as it does include the use of animals at times. However, you are never bound to make these choices, and the culture also offers a rich collection of herbal remedies. The country's history of capturing the use of alternative medicine dates back centuries to the time when it enjoyed imperial glory and when emperors were in pursuit of improved well-being to ensure longevity. Even during these early times, the nation already added a lot of value to finding doctors and medical experts who could generate records and medical records, offering a reference for future generations.

Historic records share a story that stretched over many centuries, teaching us that each dynasty had a slightly different approach to medicine and healing. During the Shennong dynasty, dating back to about 2800 B.C.E., herbs were considered to be superior, while the Shang Dynasty is the timeline many consider to be the actual start of Chinese medicine, as, during this age, herbs were often used to treat illness (Robbins, 2014). From here onwards, medicine and healing were sometimes closely linked to the spiritual world; at times, there was a greater distance between the two practices. While the approach to alternative medicine and healing may be varied over time, the one certainty we have is that alternative medicine is integral to the Chinese character and identity even today.

South and Central America

When we explore the use of herbal remedies to improve a range of ailments in South and Central America, we quickly learn that the Incan and Aztec cultures and their contribution in this regard stand integral to this kind of development. These cultures relied on herbal remedies to treat disease and injuries, but herbs also had a deeper meaning to them, as various plants played an important role in shamanism. Once again, our attention is brought to the fact that ancient cultures often relied on a spiritual aspect as the way they treated ailments while using herbs.

It is, especially, the historic records providing us with insight into the way the Aztec culture practiced herbalism that provides us with clarity on how they used herbs, religion, science, and magic to bring about healing and wellness. These records reflect methods dating back to 1522 (Lyle, 2014).

Yet, this kind of treatment isn't limited to only these cultures, as the Mayans also made an immense contribution to the development of herbal medicine. While they, too, used a holistic approach when they treated a range of health concerns, it is particularly the range of ailments they treated with herbal remedies that are quite astounding. Records indicate that they used herbs to treat coughs, bladder infections, sore throats, high blood pressure, diarrhea, backaches, and intestinal parasites rather effectively with herbal remedies (Lyle, 2014).

Africa

Africa is likely the continent where large parts of the population still rely on herbal remedies to treat a wide range of ailments. Herbs and the use of active ingredients in special plants is an ancient practice in this continent too, but due to the lack of infrastructure in large parts—as great sections of the continent are occupied by communities in rural settlements—many still turn to nature to seek healing. Here too, there is a spiritual element to healing, and, especially in the Southern parts of Africa, *sangomas*—or traditional healers—are still very active serving the communities in which they reside.

Europe

The Greek and Roman ancient civilizations stand integral in the development of herbal remedies. Their need to develop aids to treat people was emphasized by the constant attacks the barbarians would make on these ancient nations. It is especially during the years 400–1400 that Europe experienced an immense economic decline due to constant warfare (Mortlock, 2019). This situation was worsened by dire conditions caused by floods and poor living conditions that caused diseases to spread quickly. However, monasteries were more protected and they all had herbal gardens where the monks would source their herbs to blend for remedies to treat the sick. It was also a time when there was a lot of emphasis placed on the four *humors*. The term *humors* refers to the elements air, fire, water, and earth. Each of these elements symbolized a human element—for example, air symbolized blood. Treatments during this time also had a holistic approach toward healing.

The Paleolithic Period

This era is probably the oldest reference we have for understanding how people relied on plants and herbs for food and medicine. The era dates back roughly 2.5 million years ago, and, during that time, plants were a large part of the diet. The more people became familiar with plants and herbs, the better they could identify what plants work well to treat certain diseases; they were probably the first to use herbal remedies.

Considering these numerous snippets from the history of the development of herbal remedies, it is evident that across the globe, every ancient civilization relied on herbs to address health concerns and to ensure healing. Yes, there have been times when interest in herbal remedies dwindled, but times lacking interest in herbs as a way to ensure healing would always be followed by an era where interest in this regard increased once again. Currently, we are living in such an era, a time when a growing part of the global population is interested in natural ways to address health concerns without having to rely on Big Pharma.

How Does Herbal Medicine Work

This bird's eye view of the development of herbal medicine over several centuries across the globe provides certainty in knowing that there is a lot of value that we can gain from utilizing herbs in this manner. But how do herbs work? This is the vital question I want to explore before we continue any further.

Western medicine might have set itself apart from herbal medicine to such a degree that the two options we have today are almost in direct contrast with each other, and it can be easy to forget that most pharmaceutical drugs still contain elements of herbs. In some cases, as much as 50% of the composition of pharmaceutical drugs consists of either botanicals or artificially created components that resemble chemicals found in botanicals (*How Herbal Medicine Works*, n.d.).

The main difference between herbal remedies and prescription drugs is that the latter increases the concentration of the active ingredients found in herbs and is therefore stronger, delivering faster results.

Scientists in pharmaceutical labs would identify the active ingredients in plants and extract them from all the other elements, while also enhancing their strength to create a fast-acting solution. What effectively happens is that both options have the same effect on the body, but due to the higher concentration of the active ingredients in pharmaceuticals, they work much faster and bring relief quicker than when you would follow the herbal route.

So, while herbal remedies bring about gradual improvement, pharmaceuticals will create almost instant relief. The speed you can expect from pharmaceuticals makes them a desired solution in a society where we are often operating under immense stress; there is no time to be sick or to allow our bodies to recover more gradually. Hence, the largest part of the population grabs the solution that will bring them instant relief, often not even considering the price they are paying for their need to heal faster. This is a price determined by the side effects linked to many prescription drugs.

When we explored the origins of herbal medicine, it became evident that using herbal medicine required an entirely different approach than Western medicine. If I have to capture the latter in one phrase, it would probably be something like "fast-acting relief." This kind of medicine is aimed at bringing instant relief to symptoms you may experience. For example, when you have a fever, you would take paracetamol to break the fever. When you choose to rely on herbal remedies, the approach is different. In this case, you would rather simply manage your fever so that it doesn't go too high. But, the idea is to allow the body to work through the fever by itself, as it is part of the healing process. Fever serves as part of the body's natural defense as it increases the body temperature to kill off or at least slow the growth of bacteria and other harmful microorganisms.

In the same manner, the herbalist's approach towards vomiting and diarrhea is to allow it to continue while managing the state so that the patient doesn't dehydrate. Yet, this is not a comfortable state to be in, and, therefore, the approach from a Western medicine side would be to immediately stop these symptoms to get the patient to feel better soon. But, by doing so, the body is not cleansing itself from what caused it to feel this way in the first place, and now you need stronger medicine to address a concern that your body would have overcome by itself if only it was granted the time to do so.

Another major difference between Western medicine and herbal remedies is that Western medicine only focuses on the *active ingredient*—that part of the plant that helps healing—and it discards the rest of the plant. Herbal remedies often use the entire plant to offer a holistic approach, as while the other ingredients may not contribute directly to addressing a specific concern, it still supports healing.

A classic example of the link between botanicals and modern medicine is the trusted and well-known drug prescribed for cardiac disease: digitalis. The drug's name is derived from the plant species, *Digitalis Ianata*, also known as "foxglove." The ordinary plant found in many gardens is the main ingredient in prescription medication. The active ingredients in botanicals that are used in medication are called "phytochemicals," and the phytochemicals in foxglove are responsible for treating heart muscles (*How Herbal Medicine Works*, n.d.). Foxgloves and the particular way of using it is only one example of many others and the confirmation of the strong link between herbal remedies and prescription medication.

This brings us to a much deeper discussion and the topic of the next chapter: How do herbal remedies compare overall with modern medication, and why is the natural route the way to go?

Chapter 2:

Modern Medicine vs. Herbal Medicine

It is only once you have all the necessary information regarding how the pharmaceutical industry started that you'll be able to make an informed decision about whether this is the kind of industry you want to support.

The History of Big Pharma

The start of Big Pharma is undeniably linked to the name of John D. Rockefeller, an American oil magnate, and the first American to earn the title of a billionaire. Rockefeller lived during 1839–1937, and at the turn of the century, his company, Standard Oil, owned most of the oil refineries in the country.

It was during this time that scientific research had an immense breakthrough when scientists discovered that they can create a range of chemicals from oil (Kanthan, 2015). Once they've created these chemicals, they could be sold at immense prices, making them quite alluring to investment to have in your portfolio. These chemicals were perfect for the pharmaceutical industry, but there was one problem: The majority of American society was still using natural medicine. This was an obstacle in Rockefeller's way to making even greater profits. Yet, it wasn't a challenge he would be able to overcome. With the aid of his good friend, Andrew Carnegie, he managed to draft a report on the status of all medical schools and hospitals in the country, stating that these are all in desperate need of improvement. This report is widely known as the *Flexner Report*, and many consider it the foundation of modern medicine.

Due to the report, certain needs arose and Rockefeller was ready to donate over $100 million to colleges and hospitals to foot the bill for these improvements to be made. While it was an even larger investment back then than what it would be today, it was a worthy investment to make for Rockefeller, as, now, he had a foot in the door and the ability to influence what doctors across the nation would be taught. Suddenly, the message across the medical landscape echoed the same message that patented drugs are the way to go. As these medical experts were taught to believe that natural medicine is an inferior solution to what can be achieved with patented drugs, national popularity quickly swung in the favor of Rockefeller's solution, a solution that contained chemicals made from oil, an industry which he was dominating (Kanthan, 2015).

This is, of course, a much-abbreviated version of a major historical event. Yet, what it proves is that the reason why prescription drugs are preferred over natural remedies is not that it is a more effective or better solution, but quite simply because, more than a century ago, the medical society was manipulated to think this way. It is still the predominant way of thinking today.

How Big Pharma Holds Its Control

Even though this all happened almost a century ago, pharmaceutical companies still maintain this control. But how? Quite simply, they did it through a very smart multi-faceted approach.

First of all, they had to get the Food and Drug Administration's (FDA) buy-in. This they managed to corrupt it with the help of political support and, of course, large sums of money that are being allocated as sponsorships.

Similar to Rockefeller's approach, they have their fingers all over medical schools. If you teach the minds of others to practice medicine a certain way, they will likely continue to follow these teachings throughout their careers, writing an almost endless number of prescriptions for—you've guessed it—prescription drugs manufactured by pharmaceutical companies.

Then, it is also important to mention how pharmaceutical companies approach these medical experts in the field. It is a way that will keep the majority hooked for years, as pharmaceutical reps present themselves as good doers of society, the ones who are there to help and support the sick. But what are they truly selling?

Those doctors who show the motivation to search for alternatives to what they are forced to prescribe often have to face threats to their licenses for practicing medicine, as the State Medical Board is now also in the pharma camp. Thus, even if doctors may wish to use alternative medicine—even though very few have been able to escape that mindset—they are still restricted in many ways.

The latest partner in this ruthless game is the World Health Organization (WHO). See, Big Pharma notices a threat to their profits the moment it appears on the horizon, and with gained interest in alternative medicine, the need to purchase vitamins, natural remedies, and supplements increases. Now, the WHO is fulfilling its role to keep this from happening and are looking to set all kinds of restrictions in this regard in place.

While the most prestigious medical schools across the globe shift all their focus on teaching future doctors that prescription medication is the best approach to treat any health concern, they completely dismiss the vital role that healthy eating plays. Nutrition and the role food plays as a form of medicine are vastly neglected and often don't even get a mention in these classrooms. Have you ever felt the frustration of wanting to gain more information about the correct way of eating from your doctor and just not getting the answers you are looking for? That is quite simply because nutrition wasn't part of the curriculum that made them specialists in their field, and, added to that, the belief that prescription drugs are the only solution to ensure healing is drilled into them.

This is, of course, also a notion further supported by the fact that the future of any academic medical institution depends on research. Research is expensive and demands financial support. It is a situation that creates a golden opportunity for Big Pharma to expand and hold their interest, as their pockets are deep and they can manipulate the direction research takes since they foot the bill. Annually, medical research and education receive vast amounts of money from pharmaceutical companies; that is how Big Pharma controls the narrative in consulting rooms and hospitals across the globe.

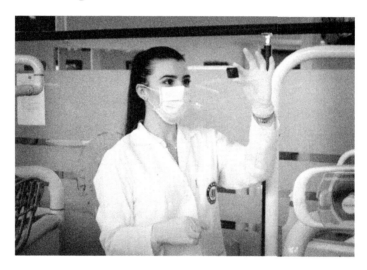

Prescription Drugs Are Addictive

Prescription drugs have many side effects. This is a statement I've made several times so far as it is such a widely known fact. However, a concern that is even much worse when it comes to many types of pharmaceuticals—and this is something far fewer people consider when they fill their prescriptions until it is too late—is that they are addictive.

Even though illegal, getting a nation hooked on pills is the most effective way to ensure that you always have a buying market.

When it comes to prescription meds that are addictive, it is especially opioids, stimulants, and antianxiety meds that top the charts. Under the umbrella of opioids, you'll find pain medication brands like Oxycontin, Norco, and Percocet. Antianxiety meds include hypnotics and sedatives like Valium, Xanax, and Ambien. Lastly, the range of stimulants can be quite extensive, and brands that are often the cause of concern are Adderall, Dexedrine, Ritalin, and Concerta (Mayo Clinic, 2022).

Other names that you may have come across are (*22 Most Dangerous*, 2017)

- Clopidogrel is a blood thinner that is widely sold as Plavix.

- Varenicline is often used to help people to quit smoking and is sold as Chantix.

- Sildenafil is more widely known as Viagra.

- Fentanyl is used to treat severe pain in patients under the brand names Abstral, Subsys, or Duragesic.

However, these names only constitute a drop in the bucket of many more drugs that are relatively freely available on the market and are highly addictive.

Side Effects of Modern Medicine

While addiction is already a major cause for concern, it is not the only risk you expose yourself to every time you fill your prescription.

No, the other challenge these pharmaceuticals pose is that they predominantly focus on treating disease and not on supporting sustained wellness.

The world of modern medicine centers around an enormous money-making game, and, therefore, there is immense competition between various manufacturers, often leaving the consumer as collateral damage in the process of generating profits. This collateral damage usually ends up leaving a path of devastation, evident in the high number of annual deaths attributed to using these drugs. Statistics indicate that prescription medication is the cause of 750,000 deaths in the States alone every year (McBride, 2022).

The States is also a nation in which some communities suffer from severe opioid addiction, causing large-scale deterioration in neighborhoods and impacting the lives of even those who are merely sharing the same space as those who are hooked on these meds.

Are we doomed? Do we have no other choice than to take such immensely high risks? These are the questions especially asked by those whose lives have been affected. Yet, you won't find the answer to these questions in the media, nor would your pharmacist or doctor provide you with an honest reply, for the truth would literally negatively impact their financial security.

Why Herbal Medicine Is the Answer

The truth is that you do have a choice. There is an alternative to medical care, and it is an alternative that doesn't pose greater threats than promises of recovery—the answer is herbal medicine.

Herbal Medicine Is Effective in Treating Medical Concerns

I've stated that many pharmaceuticals still largely contain the active chemicals found in botanicals. This is sufficient evidence proving the potent healing power found in herbs. However, it is due to a lack of knowledge regarding how to use herbs effectively that many may find that they don't get the results they've hoped for when they turn to herbal remedies. Overcoming this lack of knowledge is the focal point in Chapter 2 and the foundation of this entire book.

They Present a Safer Alternative

In their most natural form, herbs rarely pose any risks to your health and well-being, and if they do, the side effects are severely mild. It is only once the natural extracts are chemically manipulated and reconstructed in labs to extract the active ingredients and manufacture pharmaceuticals that side effects come into play.

Herbal Medicine Is Cheaper

When you rely on herbs for healing, you use a natural source that doesn't require much—if any—financial input or investment. Often, you can use herbs with minimal intervention and you can take care of this at home without any special equipment. Due to the minimal financial investment needed to use herbal medicine, it is a cheaper option compared to manufactured pharmaceuticals with high overheads and expensive price tags.

Herbs and Drugs Are Different

Alternative treatment options vary vastly from using prescription drugs, and you can't approach the two options in the same manner. Pharmaceuticals target specific symptoms or diseases, while alternative treatments follow a holistic approach and address symptoms and causes. It is a solution that may take longer to work, but it improves the state of the entire body and doesn't only focus on providing instant short-term solutions.

Herbal Remedies Create Internal Balance

Sickness or disease is often the result of an imbalance in the body. This imbalance can be caused by a deficiency or too much exposure to a certain component present in food; water; or living conditions like air pollution, stress, or malnutrition. While drugs only address the symptoms of your concern, herbal remedies restore the entire internal balance to resolve the cause of these concerns too. Some ways how herbs can do this is by addressing the causes of allergies, exhaustion, sinusitis, or even certain autoimmune concerns like arthritis. Herbs also work on your hormones and can restore hormonal imbalances, and they will always contribute to strengthening your immune system too.

The Power of Herbs Surpassed the Apothecary

Many plants have wonderful healing properties, and, in many cases, these plants are not only used for medicinal purposes but also play an important role in the culinary world. There is a huge crossover between the benefits you'll find in the herbs you eat and those you'll use for medicine. This is making it much easier to ensure sustained wellness simply by changing the way you eat.

Herbs Are Rich in Active Compounds

These plants can contain hundreds of active compounds, many of which go to waste in labs when these herbs are used in manufacturing drugs. When using herbs in their natural form, you enjoy all the benefits that these plants have to bring.

Herbal Remedies Offer a Sustainable Solution

There are large parts of the world where accessibility is limited or where communities simply can't afford Western medical care or medicine. People in these parts need and do rely on the use of alternative medicine. As they have a much richer wealth of knowledge of how to use herbs effectively, they enjoy the results they seek, proving again that herbal remedies work very well not only to treat disease but also prevent it.

Making the Shift

Are you ready to go along the road less traveled? To opt for an alternative approach to health care, an approach that is much more affordable, sustainable, and safer than what you may be used to? Transitions are normally quite hard and challenging to sustain, but when it comes to making the shift between prescription medication and using herbal medicine, it only requires changing your approach. For your entire life, you may have been made to believe that there is only one way to ensure recovery from illness or to heal wounds. Now, you know that you have an option, and it is a very attractive option to follow; you simply need to change your perspective on health care.

It will require that you gain knowledge about herbs and the plants you are about to use, as you need to be certain that you are using the correct plants, plant parts, and that you correctly prepare them. If you are making a gradual shift from the conventional to an alternative approach, it is best to do so with the support of a doctor or preferably a qualified herbalist to guide you along the way as herbs and prescription drugs can interact.

You would also need to be patient as herbal remedies take longer to bring you the results you seek, but this is not because they are any less effective, but simply because they bring healing from the inside out through a holistic approach to wellness that is lasting. One more point to keep in mind is that herbal medicine does have limitations. There are certain medical concerns that you won't be able to cure with alternative medicine. Simply think about broken bones, teeth that need to be extracted, and surgery. But, there is also a long list of medical concerns that you can very effectively treat with alternative medicine, making medical care—and especially preventative care—much more affordable and far less risky. Even when you are using herbal medicine, it is important to apply a great deal of care to what you are doing. As you may be allergic to certain compounds or elements found in food, it can be that you may show an allergic reaction toward certain plants too. Therefore, apply awareness to your use of herbal remedies and do so responsibly.

Modern Medicine vs. Herbal Medicine

Still not convinced that herbal medicine is the way to ensure lasting health and longevity, without increasing the risk of exposure to many side effects? Let's make a simple comparison between the two available treatment options.

Modern medicine is patent-protected. The consumer has little to no knowledge of the exact ingredients that go into these drugs. The names of these ingredients are printed on the labels, but it has no meaning to the average person who doesn't know these names or what their characteristics are. Knowledge about herbs and the healing properties they possess is widely available for all to learn and share.

Drugs are created according to certain scientific formulas, and the consumer—you—has to fit the mold of these drugs. When you consult a qualified herbalist, the professional will compile a treatment plant consisting of various herbs and alternative remedies to provide a holistic approach that addresses your unique concern and physical state. Herbal medicine leans itself to a patient-centric approach.

The knowledge about alternative remedies is often passed on from one generation to the other, meaning it is the knowledge that comes with an abundance of experience gained from trial and error. It is a fluid kind of knowledge that evolves based on the circumstances and unique conditions of patients. When we consider modern medicine, we can also identify a long line dating back into history. But, there are few changes, development is based only on the research done in pharmaceuticals labs, and the changing conditions of the patients are seldom considered.

At the core of modern medicine, you'll find profit margins and financial gain. Herbal medicine centers around delivering affordable, effective, holistic healing.

Can we proceed to discuss the basics of creating your home apothecary?

Chapter 3:

The Ideal Apothecary Cabinet

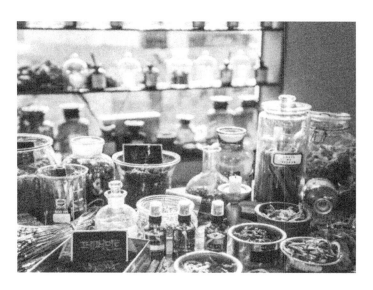

Are you excited about starting your home apothecary? I am, but before I go any further, I want to highlight that you don't have to be a qualified herbalist to be the owner of an apothecary or to rely on herbal medicine. It does help to connect with one in your area though as they will be able to answer questions that may be unique to your situation and that might not have been covered in this book. That said, I do provide quite a comprehensive guide to get you started on this journey and to bridge the gap caused by a lack of knowledge in this field.

Creating Your Herbal Apothecary

There are no set guidelines as to what exactly an apothecary should look like. We all may have different ideas of what we want to create. For some, the idea of having an antique wooden cabinet filled with little jars of dried herbs and small bottles of tinctures and oils may appear alluring, but others may prefer a version that resembles something more modern. That is perfect too; just find a storage space that is practical and suits your life and home. After all, the word *apothecary* means "storehouse" (*Creating Your Home*, n.d.), and what truly matters is what is inside of this space and your knowledge to effectively use what you have. Do take note that it is best to ensure you have plenty of storage space, even if you start out small, for the longer you are on this journey of natural healing, the larger your collection of quality herbs will grow.

That said, there are so many herbs that you can use and add to your apothecary, but as you are starting out now, I compiled a list of great herbs that will provide you with a wonderful collection to form the foundation of your apothecary. These are some of the herbs most commonly used and you can always add more along the way.

Herbs are used in several forms, and it may be best to divide the space you are going to use into the following sections:

- dried herbs

- essential oils

- tinctures

- herbal teas

By categorizing your collection of herbs this way, it is much easier to find what you are looking for when you need it.

Dried Herbs

- lavender

- peppermint

- nettle

- comfrey

- catnip

- dandelion root

- lemon balm

- chamomile

- echinacea

- tulsi

- marshmallow root

- valerian

- elderberry

- skullcap

- oat straw

- raspberry

- ashwagandha

Essential Oils

- eucalyptus

- tea tree

- lemon

- frankincense

- mandarin

- clove

- lavender

- patchouli

- blue chamomile

Basic Tinctures to Have

- reishi

- ashwagandha

- tulsi

- valerian

- Oregon grape

- burdock

- elderberry glycerite

- lemon balm

- passionflower

- echinacea

In your herbal tea storage, you'll have tea blends that will address specific concerns. Later on, I am sharing tips on how to blend a range of teas so that you always have stock that is prepared and ready to use. Typically, these blends would address concerns like colds and fevers; headaches; and allergies to support digestion or immunity.

Your list of preprepared essential-oil blends will include blends to boost your mood and immunity, reduce stress, and help with memory.

The same goes for tinctures as you'll have tinctures already blended for a specific purpose. Tincture blends are often used for cramps, menstrual pain, digestion, sleeping, and headaches.

Carrier Oils

Always also stock up on carrier oils. You'll use these oils for blending your essential oils. As essential oils and tincture can be highly concentrated, you'll have to dilute them at times; this is when you would turn to your carrier oils. Here too, you'll find a vast list of options to choose from, but the following are some of the most widely used options:

- coconut oil

- sweet almond oil

- rose hip oil

- black seed oil

- olive oil

When you purchase carrier oils, always be sure to buy quality items that you purchase from trusted and reputable providers. The last thing you would want to do is to degrade the quality of your blend because you've opted to skimp on carrier oils.

Stocking Up on Quality Items

Now you know what herbs, oils, and tinctures you need to get, but where do you source these from? Should you just visit your local health shop and make what would be quite an expensive investment? No, you'll be able to source a lot of what you need in nature. Some of these herbs, like nettles, may even be something that you used to consider to be weeds in your garden and you simply pulled them out and threw them away. So, you may even be able to get some of these items, for free, just by spending time in nature harvesting herbs. This can be a fun and exciting trip if you are well prepared.

Before heading out, be sure that you have all the tools you need to harvest herbs. Useful tools to have in your backpack would be a pair of scissors or pruning shears; a camera; a book; a pen; and a book with pictures of plants that will help to make identification easier. If you come across a plant and you are not sure whether you've identified it correctly, cut a small piece to take with you or take pictures that will help you to find it online or in plant books. Always have a bag to put your plant cutting in; I find a canvas bag works great.

Never take a plant out if you are not 100% sure that you've identified it correctly. A lot of plants look very similar, and it can be confusing to the untrained eye to make a positive identification. Therefore, it will be helpful to tag someone along who does have a better knowledge of the area you are entering.

As important as it is to identify the plants you harvest correctly, it is to identify poisonous plants. There are many poisonous plants in nature too, and you can make yourself or anyone else you try to help with your remedies very sick or worse if you've misidentified a plant. Therefore, please don't forget your book helps you to identify plants at home, especially not on your first couple of trips.

When you are in nature, remain aware of your environment and be on the lookout for possible treasures you can find. Even if you see a lot of plants that you aren't looking for, you'll get familiar with plants much faster if you are mindful on these trips. Having a sense of curiosity will also encourage you to expand on your knowledge base of what is available in your area, what plants grow in what areas, and what you can find in your region.

It is easy to get carried away, especially after harvesting your first plants, but always be considerate of the land you are exploring. If it is privately owned, check with the owner first before entering the property. Essentially, if you do enter without permission, you'll be breaking the law. Even if it is an area open to the public, you need to get permission first to harvest any plants before doing so.

Never take more than what you need. You don't want to ruin the experience for all others visiting the area after you. And, always treat nature with respect, leaving nothing behind except your admiration for the beauty and tranquility that are often part of such an expedition. Saying that, also refrain from harvesting plants in areas where there are visible signs of pollution. Plants absorb all kinds of toxins that may be present in the soil, and you don't want to carry these toxins to your apothecary. As you start to visit a specific area often, you'll start to notice what plants are seasonal or only available at certain times and which are available all year round.

Except for harvesting plants in the wild, you can also grow your own plants in your garden. Maybe you have a couple of pots that can work, raised garden beds, or any other open space that will serve as a perfectly good place to grow your own herbs. What herbs you'll be able to cultivate like this would depend on where you are located and the hardiness zones of the region. What is great about growing your own plants is that you have closer contact with them and will be able to witness all the stages they go through and be able to harvest when the time to do so is optimal.

Easy to Find Herbs in the US

Every continent consists of many regions that have different climates that are optimal for various plants to grow. It means that you'll find different plants in the United States than in Europe. The same will also be the case if you are located in the East or Africa. I'll be sharing some tips on where and what you can find in the US and United Kingdom or Europe, but if you live anywhere else, spend some time getting to know your region before stepping out to harvest.

Dandelion

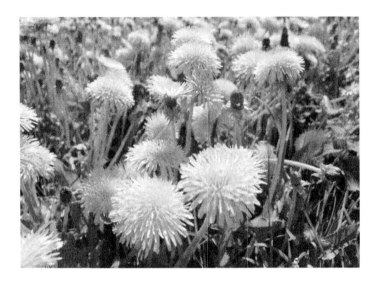

Most people are familiar with what a dandelion looks like as it is quite a common plant, often considered to be a weed. And then, of course, it also makes the magical white puffy seeds that just wait to be picked and blown into the wind with a wish. The plant does wonders to support kidney health as it is a diuretic. It also cleanses the blood and the liver of toxins. Dandelions are used to improve arthritis, skin problems, and inflammation in the joints. The leaves are edible and can add a special touch to summer salads, while the roots are used for tinctures.

Blackberries

Blackberries grow in the wild and have a beautiful deep color, are tasty, and work wonders to heal an upset stomach. The Cherokee taught modern herbalists that blackberries are also good to relieve joint pain and easing coughs. For the latter, they would mix blackberries with maple syrup or honey to create a very tasty coughing syrup. It is not only the berries that are helpful but also the leaves. By chewing the leaves, you can improve bleeding gums.

Motherwort

Motherwort helps to soothe your nerves and serves as a great aid to reduce stress, making it a wonderful addition to any apothecary. It also relieves heart palpitations and is an effective tonic for women. The plant is also effective to treat various concerns related to fertility and the reproductive system, from improving fertility to bringing your menstrual cycle back on track.

Sage

Sage is no stranger in the kitchen, as this herb is widely considered to offer rich flavors to a range of dishes. Yet, we shouldn't limit this beautiful plant to the kitchen. It is also a helpful aid to treat spasms, colds, and flu, as well as stomach cramps.

Lemon Balm

Lemon balm may not be as well known as sage when it comes to cooking, but it is not unknown either. The plant's leaves have a refreshing aroma when crushed.

These leaves also make the perfect bedtime tea that will help to overcome insomnia. Cold sores can be painful and something to feel self-conscious about, but you can quickly address this concern with lemon balm and may experience even better results than from an over-the-counter (OTC) alternative.

Lavender

This is, of course, another household name across many parts of the world. Lavender is amazing to smell and beautiful to look at. It is also one of those plant species that has quite a bit of variety as there are many cultures available. While the scent of lavender attracts bees, it repels most other insects, so you can rub these leaves on your arms and legs when out camping or sitting around the campfire. If you were too late with your lavender leaves and were bitten by insects, lavender will improve the itching, as it also offers relief to minor burns and rashes.

Prickly Pear

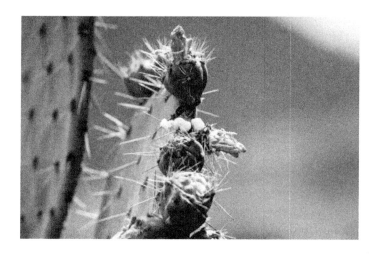

The prickly pear cactus can be found in several warmer parts of the US. The fruits can be eaten, but it is far more than merely a snack. Native Americans would make tea from the plant to treat urinary tract diseases and they would use a poultice made from mature pads of the plant to treat burns, boils, and open wounds. Researchers now also found that the plant is an effective treatment for cholesterol, and can aid in preventing heart disease and type 2 diabetes (ANNE, 2017).

Weeping Willows

You'll find these trees with their hanging branches near water sources as they demand high water consumption. Boil about a handful of these leaves in a cup of water for at least ten minutes and allow it to cool down. Dip a clean cloth in the water and use it to treat ulcers, boils, and abscesses. It can also come to your aid if diarrhea is the problem you are facing. Simply scrape some of the bark off the branches and soak it in hot water. Sip away on this drink every two hours and your problem will clear up soon.

Echinacea

Over recent years, "echinacea" became a more common term as more people realize its contribution to combating colds and flu. Typically, you would make tea from the plant's leaves or roots and have a few regular sips. The active ingredients support your immune system. While it may not stop you from getting sick altogether, it does ensure colds are less severe and it shortens the recovery time. As the active ingredient fights off fungi, it also clears up yeast infections and minimizes the chances of your infection returning.

These 10 examples merely serve as an indication of how available these plants are and how easy it is to make your own herbal remedies. Depending on in which area you stay, these plants are widely available as they grow wild in nature. It also means that these plants bring you affordable health care.

Easy to Find Herbs in the UK and Europe

The UK and Europe have similar weather conditions and climates, and, therefore, there are a lot of plants that are easily available in both locations. The following are all herbs you'll find with little effort if you reside in either.

Sting Nettle

Have you ever felt the sting of this nettle? It is often the case that you may not even see the plant and innocently reach for something else, and then it gets you. Sadly, the sting is also the reason why many wouldn't even consider the health properties of this plant, and there are many you can enjoy. Sting nettle leaves can improve allergy symptoms and the latest research breakthrough indicates that these plants can even help as a treatment for Alzheimer's disease.

Evening Primrose

Typically, you would harvest the plant's leaves to make oil. The oil has wonderful properties that aid in pain relief and it speeds up healing. Taking this oil regularly also eases the symptoms of menopause.

English Marigolds

It is hard to miss these with their bright orange flowers that adorn many gardens across the UK. But, the marigold is not just a pretty sight to look at. Dry the flowers of the plant and rub them onto stings and bites; it will reduce the swelling and improve the pain. Fresh flowers can also be used to treat skin problems.

Feverfew

Do you suffer from migraines? These severe headaches can bring your entire life to a standstill, but feverfew may just be the answer you were hoping for. The best part is that the plant contains all the active ingredients you need to address the symptoms and causes of migraines when you are suffering from one and by taking it regularly, you can even reduce your chances of getting them so often.

Ladies Mantle

There is a reason why this plant, which is mostly found in Northern UK, contains the word "ladies" in its name. It is part of the rose family and is mostly used to treat ailments that ladies experience. It is also great for relieving muscle spasms and can even be used to treat open wounds and cuts.

Elder

Elder flowers add a tasty flavor to cordials but it is also antiseptic and anti-inflammatory. The plant was trusted in ancient times as a treatment for arthritis and colds and relieving inflammation and pain caused by a range of other concerns.

How to Harvest Herbs

Harvesting can be a challenge, not because anything is challenging to it but simply because many—especially those new to building their apothecary—don't know how to do it. It can be easy to get carried away with the excitement of hunting for the perfect plants, being sure that you've found what you are looking for, and then having no idea what to do with it.

Harvesting herbs doesn't mean that you rip the entire plant out of the soil. There are many herbs from which you'll only use the aerial parts and then simply have to cut what you need and leave the rest of the plant intact.

Harvesting Aerial Parts of the Herb

The term *aerial* refers to everything visible above the soil; this can be leaves, stems, and—if in bloom— flowers too. By following these steps, you can be sure that you harvest exactly what you need and will leave a strong plant behind that can recover quickly.

When cutting these parts, go down about a quarter or even a third from the top of the plant and only cut these parts. Make sure that you still leave a couple of stems intact at their full length. By doing so, the plant will recover much faster. It is always best to cut these stems just above the leaf nodes.

This is the preferred way to harvest aerial parts off a plant. But, if you simply grab a bunch of leaves in your hands and just chop them off, you'll still get what you need and the plant will survive.

But what about plants that don't have stems, like parsley? Here, you'll grab a handful of leaves and chop them right above the surface, but make sure that you leave at least a third of the plant still intact. Follow this method unless the plants you harvest have thick stems, like lemongrass. Then, you would only snip away the softer leafy tops.

Getting Quality Bark

The best time to harvest bark is when there is more sap in the tree, but the leaves haven't started to branch out. Usually, this happens in early spring. The second best time is autumn once the leaves change their color and the tree begins to shed them in preparation for winter.

Keep in mind that a tree is alive and never peel the bark straight off the tree. This will leave damage that it will struggle to recover from. The correct method is to prune a branch first, the best way is to aim for twigs that are roughly 1 ½ inches thick. If you use young branches like these, you spare yourself time and effort, as there is no need to peel the outside bark first and the young branches will quickly be replaced by new branches.

The way you are going to cut these branches when pruning them will depend on the kind of tree you are working with. When you want the tree to grow bushier, you can make a heading cut above the node. If you want to thin it out, rather make a thinning cut and cut down the entire branch right at the trunk of the tree.

If an older tree has to be cut down or has fallen down, you can use the bark of the entire tree, but you'll have to remove the outer bark first. The bark on the trunk and thicker branches can be very rough, so even if all the bark is available, maybe just use the young bark on thin branches and twigs.

Harvesting young bark is easy. Just rip off any leaves and then use a peeler to scrape slices of bark off the twig or branch. If the bark is too thick for a peeler, you can also use a knife. Sometimes, bark can be very hard to peel as it is stuck to the inner section of the branch, so you can bash it a little to make it softer. A hammer will work, but a stone can be as effective too.

Remember that bark has a high tannin content, and you'll need to add glycerin to your tinctures if that is what you plan to do with your harvest. A great measure is a 1:9 ratio for the glycerin you need to add.

Flowers and Buds, What to Take

These are very easy to harvest. Simply use your nails or, if you prefer, clippers to trim off the flowers with the entire bud intact. Mostly, you'll want to have the entire flower, but you may also have to remove the petals sometimes. For example, when you harvest chamomile, you'll use the entire flower, but for dandelions, you'll have to rip the petals off.

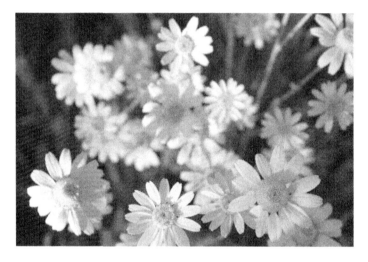

Flowers dry best when they are laid out in a single layer. They can dry naturally, but if you stay in a more humid area, you might want to invest in a dehydrator.

Roots—Getting in Underneath the Surface

The best times for root harvesting are spring and autumn. Loosen the soil a bit before cutting off a section with a sharp spade. If you have a hori hori, you can use that too. Shake off as much dirt as you can before washing off the rest of the dirt under running water. You must clean the roots completely. Fresh roots are the best to use, so cut them into pieces. Alternatively, if you want to store the roots, you have to dry them first. Here too, a dehydrator may come in handy, or you can put them in the oven for a bit to dry out at a temperature of 100–120 °F.

Once your harvest is complete, use it as quickly as possible for your tinctures. Fresh is the best, but you can also dry them. Always just remember to ensure that your plant parts are clean and don't contain any bugs or dirt.

Alternative Sources for Seeds and Herbs

The quality of the content of your apothecary would depend on the quality of the ingredients you use when mixing teas, tinctures, or even essential-oil blends. As you get more comfortable with identifying the different types of plants and how to distinguish between what are good-quality herbs and seeds and which are of inferior quality—many providers don't offer premium products even though they ask a similar price for their product—it would be best to rely only on trusted and reputable providers. There are several such suppliers available online that enable you to source any herb or seed you would need, even if the plant doesn't grow naturally in your environment.

I highly recommend the following online herb wholesalers, and I can state that you can safely purchase what you need from them and be sure that you'll get quality seeds and herbs for your money.

Recommended U.S. Providers

Readers based in the US can shop from these four herb wholesalers with an absolute peace of mind.

#1 Frontier Co-Op

You'll find Frontier Co-Op at the following website: www.frontiercoop.com. The co-op is based on its 56-hectare premises with 145,000-square foot storage outside of Norway, Iowa. The co-op has 40,000 members who are all active in the business, and, therefore, they can offer their clients a comprehensive selection of herbs and organic products. The brand's values reflect its commitment to quality products and to the environment. They are constantly promoting a message of a strong environment and social commitment.

#2 Mountain Rose Herbs

The supplier is committed to fair trade and also has the necessary certification in this regard. The wholesaler is based near Eugene, Oregon, and they offer online shopping on their website: www.mountainroseherbs.com. Their selection of premium products includes teas, essential oils, herbs, and spices. Mountain Rose Herbs is committed to organic agriculture and sustainability.

#3 Oregon's Wild Harvest

As the name states, this wholesaler is based in Redmond, Oregon. What started out as a husband-and-wife team grew into a much larger undertaking with a team that now has more than 40 farmers involved in the business. Their secret to success is their commitment to ensuring they use only plants that grow in healthy soil to provide their clients with nothing but the best. They are open to online purchases and you'll find they have a vast range of products on offer at www.oregonswildharvest.com

#4 Pacific Botanicals

The wholesaler is based in the Applegate Valley near Grants Pass, Oregon, and they are a certified grower of medicinal herbs. This is the kind of certification they could only earn through their consistent commitment to organic farming and by employing the correct methods from feeding the soil with approved nutrients to saving seeds from plants. While the brand grows a lot of its herbs itself, they also rely on other organic farmers globally to grow herbs that don't flourish in their specific microclimate. You'll find them at www.pacificbotanicals.com.

Other Sources to Explore

I—and many others—consider these four wholesalers to be the very best providers in the United States. That said, though, several other brands are also good, and you can order from them, too, with confidence. I am referring here to Mary's Heirloom Seeds, Strictly Medicinal Seeds, Johnny's Selected Seeds, and Herbal Academy.

Recommended U.K. and European Providers

Here, I can recommend three top providers you can trust when you purchase your herbs.

#1 Sarah Raven

Sarah Raven is the go-to supplier for those new to herbalism, as well as those who have years of experience in the field. Their online store—found at www.sarahraven.com—stocks everything you can possibly need to get your garden started and to maintain it in optimal condition, from gardening kits to seeds, bulbs, or plants. Sarah Raven even offers gifts, or you can attend one of their very insightful courses on the farm in East Sussex. The brand is committed to being responsible for the environment and society. The fact that they've won the Best Gardening Brand Award three years in a row is, of course, also a testimony to the excellence you can expect from Sarah Raven.

#2 Herbal Haven

Herbal Haven is a family business that has been around for two decades. They offer their clients an immense range of herbs for medicinal and culinary use. The family serves their clients with their wealth of knowledge and offers guidance to ensure that you give your plants the best care they need. They are committed to providing only strong plants that have been grown in a natural environment. The brand's commitment to farming along with the environment—without causing it any harm—is evident in its special range of herbs for bees. You'll find their online store at www.herbalhaven.com. Alternatively, you can pay them a visit at their farm near Saffron Walden, Cambridge.

#3 Nicky's Nursery

Are you looking for pot herbs, culinary herb seeds, ornamental herbs, dye plants, Chinese herbs, or plants for companion planting? You'll find it all at Nicky's Nursery located near Broadstairs, Kent; or, you can shop online at www.nickys-nursery.co.uk. The brand's herb collection is so vast that you'll be able to find quality seeds for any kind of herb you are looking for.

If you don't find what you are looking for with any of these three providers, you can still place your order with any of the brands I've identified as premium providers in the US.

It is a wonderfully exciting feeling to get your apothecary going and to harvest and plant your own herbs. Another joy is, of course, seeing how your plants grow as you nurture them with care.

Chapter 4:

Herbalism at Home—Getting Started

Harvesting herbs sure adds a fun and exciting appeal to herbalism as an alternative approach to healing, but it has certain limitations too. You may be living in an urban setting and getting to a natural environment where you'll find that an abundance of plants growing wild is just not an option. Or, you may be so severely time-restricted that you just can't find the time for such an excursion. In no way should the lack of access to herbs and plants growing wild in nature keep you from making the healthier choice when it comes to healing and health care.

The alternative is, of course, to grow your own herbs. Doing this is also a wonderful experience, as you can see how the plants you'll use grow through all their stages. You'll be able to nurture them to grow into an optimal state and have the pleasure of harvesting from when they are in a peak condition. But, the best part is that these plants will be easily accessible and getting the herbs you need will require minimal time.

Step-by-Step Guide to Growing Herbs at Home

Starting any garden at home may be daunting, especially if you have no experience with gardening. It is even more so the case when you are planting a functional garden, meaning you want to harvest produce—in this case, herbs. However, the steps to creating an herb garden are not complex to follow at all.

Shop for Quality

Whether you are going to buy seeds or seedlings, always buy quality items. There are a lot of online providers available and you may see pictures of the healthiest plants on their sites, but they by no means serve as an indication of the quality of plants or seedlings you'll receive from them. So, always do your research and read reviews of what other clients say about the supplier and the quality of the products they offer before making your payments.

The second point to consider is that you don't have to start with it all at once. I recommend that you start small and decide on three or maybe four different herbs to plant. First, find your green fingers with these before expanding your herb garden. Some plants are easy growers and the way they grow will encourage even the most inexperienced gardener to continue on this journey, so shop for these plants. Great options to start with are basil, mint, or parsley.

Sourcing Soil

The most important thing to understand about soil is that it may appear to be dead, but it is very much alive. Soil contains a lot of microorganisms that need an optimal habitat to flourish. These organisms help to break down organic material to release nutrients into the soil that plants need to grow. They are also responsible for improving the structure of the soil and for creating air pockets that prevent the soil from becoming too compact, straining root growth. Most herbs need soil that has great drainage. You should be able to find quality soil at the same supplier of your plants and seeds without having to pay too much for it.

Finding the Perfect Place to Plant or Sow

Where are you going to plant your seedlings or seeds? If you want to take up a corner of your garden for this, choose a spot where there is sufficient sunlight and preferably morning sun. Herbs do need a lot of sunlight, but the afternoon sun tends to be much harsher on plants, and, if possible, try to minimize this kind of exposure. You can also plant your herbs in pots or planters to place on a window sill or on a balcony. If you choose this option, always settle for pots that offer enough soil depth to give the roots space to grow.

Ensure that there is enough space between the different plants so that they can branch out. While you should secure that every plant is firmly placed in the soil, it is best not to compress the soil too much.

Watering

Regularly check on the dampness of your soil. Even if the soil is still damp deep within the pot but dry on the surface, it is time to water your plants again. When watering, it is better to give your plants little water more often than to give them too much at once. Plants can be overwatered and then they will drown.

Germination

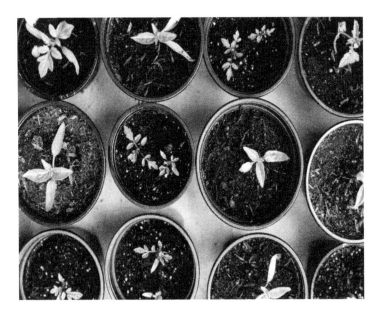

For the first couple of days, even sometimes a week or two, you may not see any life in your pots after sowing seeds. Just have patience, as the germination of seeds can take a bit of time and some seeds take even longer to germinate than others. It is a great joy when you do start to see the first little green heads showing up above the surface. The packets in which your seeds come will

state on the back how long you should expect to wait to
see any growth.

Harvesting

After germination, it may take several more weeks or
even months until you'll be able to harvest. Until then,
you can enjoy watching your plants grow. Harvesting
should be done gently, and always harvest only what
you need, even if you harvest from your own garden.

Gardening Tips

Gardening requires a certain investment of your money
and, even more so, time. Therefore, you will want to
have an optimal return on your investment. Having to
deal with an herb garden that is just not performing as
you've envisioned it can be frustrating. This is especially
the case if you are new to herb gardening, as you can
see that something is not well with your garden but
don't have the knowledge or expertise to identify
exactly what it is you need to address.

The following tips will help to realize your gardening
dreams so that you can harvest healthy herbs for your
apothecary.

Choose Plants That Flourish in Your Area

What are the herbs other people are planting in your area? The US is a vast continent and across the States, there are many areas that all have different climates. In gardening, these different climate zones are called "hardiness zones." Hardiness zones are mostly linked to the temperature variances any region would experience. For example, Texas is located in a hardiness zone of 8, meaning the minimum temperatures common for Texas range within 10–25 °F. Nebraska is in a hardiness zone of 4–5. So, here, the minimum temperature can be as low as -30 °F (The National Gardening Association, n.d.).

These temperatures determine how long your planting season would be but also what plants will do best in that area. Don't get ahead of yourself by just purchasing all the herbs you think you may like if you're not sure whether they'll grow in your climate. Rather, first explore a hardiness map and see what plants will do well in your region and when you need to plant them.

Keeping the external factors in consideration is of far greater importance when you are planning to cultivate herbs in your garden. Plants that grow inside your home are more protected against the cold, but you still need to be sure that they'll get enough sunlight.

My suggestion is to compile a list of all the herbs you would like to have at home. Then, research your hardiness zone to see what plants grow naturally in your surroundings. Scrap all the herbs from your list that don't comply with these requirements. Consider the time of the year and whether it would be a good time to plant herbs straight away; maybe you'll have to wait until it is warmer. Now, you can pick three or four herbs to get your garden started.

Harvest the Seeds of Annuals

Most herbs are annual plants and you would need to plant them every year. With most herbs, it is also the leaves that you want to harvest. Therefore, leave the plants alone, even after you've harvested them, until they make seeds. Harvest these seeds and keep them in a cool dry place to replant next year.

Prepare the Soil

If you stay in an area with very cold winters and, possibly, snowfall, it is important to let the soil warm up and to prepare it before planting. You can work in some compost and work the soil a bit to loosen it up before planting.

Tips for the Urban Gardener

An urban garden can be a beautiful space and it is relatively easy to grow a garden in your home or on a balcony. Herbs don't require a lot of space, and you don't need large quantities of herbs to make your herbal remedies. It means that even if you have minimal space, you can still grow a garden very effectively.

It will also help to explore your neighborhood a little to see if there are any urban or rooftop gardens where you can get involved. Across most cities, there are many gardening groups, and you only need to find the right one for you. These gardening spaces offer plenty of planting space for you to grow and share your herbs.

If the only available space is indoors, then that is also fine. Many seedlings do better indoors anyway.

The Tools You'll Need

Gardening on this small scale doesn't require a lot of tools. But, you'll need suitable containers to grow these herbs in; a soil knife or hori hori; a small spade; a watering can or hose; and then the soil and seeds.

An Easy Guide to Grow the Most Popular Herbs at Home

So far, I've shared some of the most basic steps to getting your garden growing. But, you'll soon realize that every type of herb is unique and can be described as having a unique personality. They have certain ways they prefer to be treated and, by giving them what they want, you'll enjoy a greater yield. I wanted to explore some of the herbs you can easily grow at home, not only to provide you with a more comprehensive reference of what you need to do but also because there are some herbs on this list that gardeners don't even realize they can grow at home with great ease.

Coriander

Coriander grows best in full sun with its roots in soil offering great drainage. It is an herb that you can easily grow from seeds. Crushing the seeds just a little before placing them in the soil will help them to germinate faster. You can sow these seeds directly into the soil of the container you want them to grow. But, if you choose to first let them sprout and then replant the seedlings, use a multi-cell tray as their roots grow quite long and are facing damage risk when you remove them from the tray.

As coriander likes sunlight, you'll have to water them regularly to ensure that the soil stays damp. Damp soil will keep the plant from making premature flowers and shortening your harvest period. Coriander will grow better if you add a little liquid seaweed to the soil, and it doesn't need anything else.

Dill

Sow your dill seeds between April and July if you are located in the Northern hemisphere. Depending on how early you've sown these seeds, you'll be able to harvest them between June and October. Dill seeds are very small, so it is best to sow them directly into the pot or planter where you want them to grow, but you can also sow them in trays and replant them into larger pots. Take care not to put the seeds any deeper than ½ inch underneath the surface. By sowing your dill in intervals during the sowing season, you'll be able to harvest your dill for much longer.

Dill needs quite a bit of water, and by clearing your pot regularly from weeds, you'll minimize any competition for the plant to get the water it needs. Usually, dill doesn't need any feeding, but the plant is quite flimsy, so you may have to support it just a little with a cane.

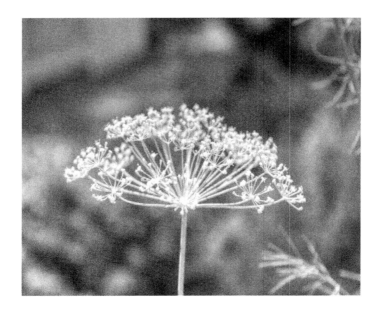

Mint

There are so many different types of mint that you can plant, and I recommend that you choose more than one to add variety to your apothecary. You can harvest mint from May to November, as it has quite a long harvesting season.

Mint is quite a hardy plant, which is good in the sense that it can survive even less favorable conditions, but it also means that it will compete with other plants, so it is best to keep it in a pot. Even though it is a perennial, it will benefit from fresh soil annually. The best way to grow mint is to get root cuttings or young plants. Even though it is hardy, plant your mint where it will have some shade as the leaves can get burn marks if it is exposed to too much sun. The plant does need to have its roots moist and the soil must have great drainage and contain sufficient levels of nutrients.

Basil

Basil is an annual plant, and sowing their seeds from February to July will ensure that you have a great harvest between June and September. It is a highly fragrant plant synonymous with many Italian recipes. Once seedlings are big enough, you can plant them in individual pots. Basil doesn't need lots of water, and if its roots are growing in moisture, your plant will underperform. When it comes to harvesting, it is best to pick only the leaves you need rather than cutting off whole pieces of the plant.

Tarragon

Tarragon doesn't produce many flowers or seeds, and the most effective manner to plant it is by using root cuttings. It is a perennial and is quite hardy, especially when it comes to sun exposure, but it needs protection from the wind and extreme cold. The soil must have great drainage and be very fertile, so it wants regular composting.

Chives

Chives grow from seeds and they come back every year. Once you've planted chives once in a pot or bedding, you can be sure that they will sprout again the very next year. That said, even though chives do well in pots, it does even better when you have it growing in beddings.

Once your chive seedlings are about 2 inches tall, you can replant them to where you want them to grow. This needs to be a spot that has well-drained, fertile soil and is either in full sun or some shade. You need to keep the soil damp and therefore regular watering is necessary.

Thyme

You can harvest thyme all year round even though the planting season is only between March to May and again from September to November. It is a fragrant herb playing an important role in many recipes. Thyme does well in a sunny spot as exposure to heat brings its aromatic oils to the surface, but it does need a lot of water until the plant is well established. Once your plant has reached this stage, it will need far less water and will survive most dry conditions.

There are also several types of thyme to choose from; some of them are so hardy, they'll even grow in cracked paving. That said, some types of thyme are far more fragile, and you would have to provide an indoor space during the coldest months of the year. Thyme seeds can be a bit of a challenge to get growing. So, save yourself the trouble and just buy seedlings as these you'll find everywhere. Add compost to the soil before planting, as thyme needs many nutrients.

Parsley

Parsley is a biennial plant, but it is best to give it the same treatment as you would an annual. It needs a spot where there is enough sun but has partially shaded areas too. The soil must have sufficient drainage. Sow these seeds no deeper than ½ inch below the surface and about 15 inches apart from each other. Keep in mind that parsley seeds can take as long as 6 weeks before they germinate, but if you sow them in intervals, you'll have enough parsley to harvest over time. Once your seedlings are about 3 inches tall, you can plant them into bigger pots about 7 inches apart. The best time to sow these seeds is between March and June and you'll be able to harvest between June and October.

Sorrel

Sorrel can grow from seeds, but because it is a perennial, you'll be able to plant root cuttings too. Make sure that you get your seeds or new root cutting in the soil between March and June; harvest time takes place between May and September. It needs soil with high water retention and does well in full sun or partially shaded spots. Water your sorrel often enough to prevent it from making seeds too soon. Sorrel dies back a bit during winter time, but you can cut the dead leaves off and divide the plant in spring to ensure another great yield.

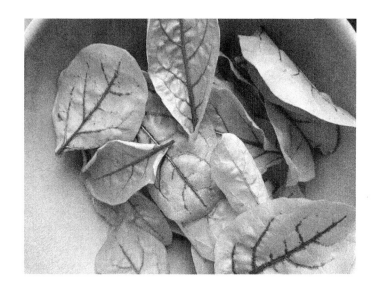

Bay

Bay trees can be a bit more tricky to care for as they need full sun but also sufficient protection. These trees need soil that is rich in nutrients and well drained. If your hardiness zone is one of the ones with more extreme cold weather, it will be beneficial to plant your bay in a pot, making it easier to bring the plant indoors to shield it from extreme cold. You can harvest the leaves off the tree during the entire year to dry them out for storage or to use them fresh.

Chervil

Chervil is related to parsley and tastes like aniseed. The plant is quite hardy and can easily grow outside as it is an annual. The seeds also germinate quickly, meaning you can sow them successively to extend your harvest. Chervil needs full sun or partial shade and well-drained soil to flourish. The plant grows only about 30 inches high and can be planted in pots.

Sage

Sage has beautiful leaves of dark green with a purple tone. You'll be able to harvest all year long from this plant, which comes as an annual and biennial plant, and both grow well from seeds. Then, there is also perennial sage for which you would need to get young plants. Sage does very well in a pot, but be sure to place your pot in direct sunlight, as here too, sunlight brings the plant's fragrant oil to the surface. When you have a perennial sage, it is best to prune the plant slightly after it flowers; this will prevent it from becoming too woody. It is also best to take some cuttings from your perennial sage to be sure you have more strong plants when others die.

Shiso

Shiso, or Chinese basil, has beautiful purple leaves and brings an amazing flavor to many meals. It is a relatively hardy plant that does well in drained soil and full sunlight. Don't overwater your shiso as it only needs water when the soil is dry. The plant grows well in sandy and clay soil. The only time that your shiso is really at risk is during cold weather, and then you would need to offer it some protection. These can be planted in pots and they grow to be about 15 inches tall.

Garlic

There are several types of garlic, but they can all be divided into two groups: *hard-neck plants*, where the garlic bulb has a very distinct neck section, and *soft-neck plants* without a neck. Garlic does well in pots, but they are vulnerable to root fungi, meaning you need to use soil that drains well. In fact, the best solution would be to refrain from using soil at all and to rather opt for a soil-less potting mixture as this would provide a light enough structure to prevent this disease.

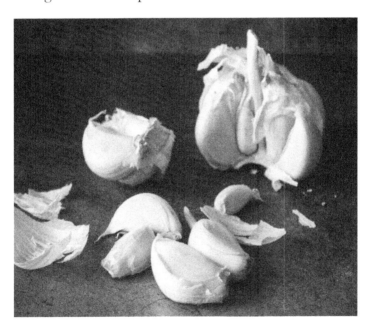

To plant garlic, break the bulb into cloves. Do not remove the papery outer layers and only plant the larger cloves. Garlic should be planted with the pointy side of the clove facing up and not too close to the brim of the pot. There should be about 1 inch of soil on top of these cloves. Garlic can sprout and then die down if the weather conditions are too cold, but it will sprout again. Your pot should be placed in a sunny place where it will get about 6 hours of sunlight. While you would need to keep the soil moist at all times, it is important that there is great drainage and sufficient sun to prevent rot.

Garlic that grows indoors will only bring you sprouts. You can trim these when they reach a length of 4 inches, but if you want bulbs, you'll have to plant them outdoors.

Echinacea

Echinacea is a popular ingredient in herbal medicine due to the many health properties of the plant, but it also makes a flower that can add color to your garden. Echinacea is a perennial that is perfectly capable of surviving dry conditions and does well in pots. Make sure that you have sufficient drainage in the pot by adding a gravel layer of about 2 inches at the bottom and drilling drainage holes in the base. Next, you'll need to fill the pot halfway up with fast-draining soil and compress this down to remove air pockets. Place the young plant into the pot and fill it up to the brim with soil. The plant likes the morning sun and more shade in the afternoon. When watering the pot, take care not to splash water on the plant itself. Remove any dead flowers when you see them to redirect energy toward the healthy flowers. It is best to fertilize the plant about every 10 days and after 3–4 years; replant the pot; and give it fresh soil.

Rosemary

Rosemary can be harvested all year round, but the best times to plant it are between March and May and then again from September to November. Rosemary is quite resistant to frost, but a combination of cold and excessive moisture can kill younger plants. So, place your rosemary in a sheltered spot with plenty of sunlight. The best way to plant rosemary is from young plants. It requires minimal maintenance, but enough fertilizer during its growing season will encourage it to do well. You can harvest rosemary as you need it. If you take proper care of your plant, you'll have rosemary for many years to come.

Cayenne Pepper

These peppers can be planted in your garden if your minimum temperatures aren't too low; otherwise, keep them in pots indoors. Cayenne peppers grow from seeds that you can plant directly into a container filled with soil that is light and offers great drainage. Place gravel at the bottom of your pot and then fill it with soil to about 1 ½ inches from the top. Water the soil and allow it to drain for 24 hours before planting your seeds. Seeds should be no deeper than ¼ inch below the surface. These peppers need about 6 hours of sunlight daily. Cayenne peppers shouldn't go dry, but it is also important not to overwater them. If the top inch of the surface is dry, it is best to give them some water. If you want cayenne peppers that have more burn to them, you need to stop watering them once the peppers start to ripen.

Turmeric

Did you know that you can grow turmeric at home? Turmeric can grow very well in pots of about 10–14 inches deep. As you'll be harvesting the roots of the plant, it is important to have enough soil depth to ensure a healthy root system develops underneath the surface. The best time to plant turmeric is during spring and summer, and then you'll be planting rhizome cuttings. If you have a large piece of rhizome, you can always break it into smaller bits and then place these about 2 inches below the surface. Make sure that you leave the buds on the rhizome facing upwards. Turmeric does especially well in warmer climates, and it needs soil with a high organic-content level. The only time when turmeric can become vulnerable is when the soil gets too dry. So, make sure that you keep the soil moist throughout the year.

In colder parts, it is important to protect the plant in cool weather, and you may have to bring the pot inside. Never prune the plant, but if there are dry leaves, you can remove these. Your turmeric should be ready to harvest after about 10 months of planting. The plant's leaves and stem will become dry. Remove the plant from the pot and harvest as many roots as you need. Replant the remaining roots in the soil for your next harvest.

Ginger

Ginger can be grown from the roots of the plant. You'll be able to find these at your local nursery. You must soak your gingerroot in hot water overnight before planting it as this will help the root to grow. As the gingerroot grows horizontally, you only need a shallow pot to grow ginger at home. The soil needs to contain lots of minerals and nutrients and have lots of drainage. Plant your roots 1 inch below the surface, but place it with the eye-bud side pointing upwards. The pot doesn't need to have a lot of sunlight, but it needs to stay relatively warm. Usually, within 3 weeks after planting, you'll see that the shoot is breaking through the surface, and only a couple of months later, you can harvest your gingerroots. When you do, take as much as you need and replant the rest of the roots so they can continue to grow.

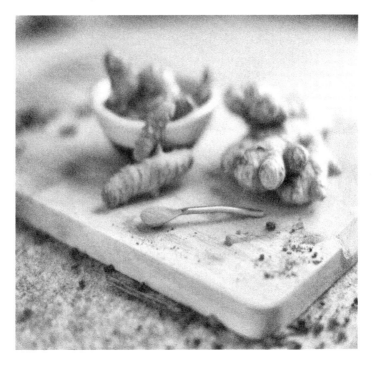

Even though this is quite a mouthful, there are even more options to choose from to add to your garden at home. To enjoy optimal results from your herb garden by harvesting from plants that bring in high yields, it would be beneficial to research the exact requirement of the herb you want to add to your collection. A great place to do this is to study an herbal encyclopedia, as this will help you to take optimal care of every herb in your garden.

Storing and Drying Herbs

It is wonderful to have fresh herbs to work with, but you'll want herbs for your herbal remedies around the year. Through proper drying and storing, you can be sure to have healthy ingredients to use in your herbal remedies.

You'll use dry herbs when making tea blends, infusing oils, and making tinctures. The greatest threats to impact the quality of your stored herbs are sunlight, moisture, oxygen, and heat. Also, remember that herbs have a storage life, and, at some point, you'll need to discard the herbs you haven't used. Even though fresh herbs are always the most potent, there are several ways to ensure your dried herbs contain all the goodness you need from them. Each of the following tips is directly linked to preventing exposure to any of the threats I've mentioned.

Store Them Whole

It is best to dry and store your herbs whole. It may be tempting to grind or chop your herbs into smaller pieces to speed up the drying process, but it is not a great idea. When you store your herbs in a whole form and only grind them down when you need them, you can be sure that it will contain more goodness.

Herbs Must Be Completely Dry

Before placing your herbs in storage, check that they have dried completely. If you are going to put herbs in a jar or any other airtight container while they still contain some moisture, it can cause mold. The most effective dryness test is to see how well the plants crumble when you rub them between your fingers. If it doesn't have a crispy feel or crumbles easily, it isn't completely dry yet. You can use a drying screen to dry your herbs. If you are going to dry herbs regularly, it will be beneficial to buy a dehydrator; dehydrators may also be the best option if you stay in a humid environment.

Avoid Sunlight

Don't underestimate the damaging effect that sunlight can have on your herbs. Sunlight robs your herbs of all the goodness they contain, and, therefore, it is best to store your herbs in dark-colored glass bottles. If you can't find these, place them in a cabinet and only take the herbs out when you need them.

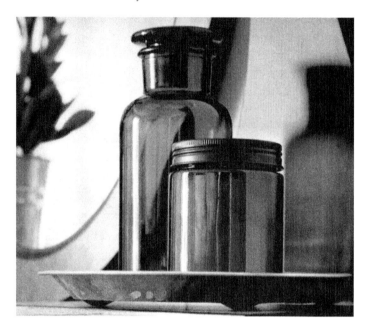

Keeping Oxygen Away

We need oxygen to breathe and live, but oxygen exposure can also lead to degradation in organic material. Therefore, the more oxygen exposure your herbs will have, the greater the impact of this exposure will be. The best way to store your herbs is in glass containers that offer an airtight seal. Avoid plastic containers simply because plastic contains so many chemicals, and, over time, your herbs may get contaminated due to direct exposure to these chemicals.

Keep Them Cool

Where are you planning to set up your apothecary? The most common place to store pharmaceuticals is in the bathroom cabinet or in the kitchen. Ironically, these two rooms are the worst places to keep your herbal remedies. Both rooms tend to get very warm and have a high moisture content. Identify a room in your home where it is cool and dry. It is often the case that bedrooms meet the standards for storing herbs as they tend to be cooler rooms and there is limited moisture exposure.

Add a Date to the Label

When you are storing your herbs, it is important that you clearly mark what is in the jar as it may become confusing when you have several jars of dried leaves that all look similar. Once you've added quite several dried herbs to your collection, it will be hard to determine what they are just by smelling them. Trying to find the one you are looking for will be a time-consuming process, but it can also be risky to confuse one herb for another.

Just as important is adding a date to each label. The date should either be the date when you harvested the herb or the date of purchase.

Below is more beneficial information to include on the label:

- the name of the herb and its botanical name

- the harvest or purchase date

- the expiration date of the herb

In general, herbs will last one to two years, but it is not a case of them going rotten after this time nor of turning bad. They just become far less potent, and you won't be able to enjoy the benefits you should from them. Once herbs have been powdered, the expected lifespan is cut in half.

Alternative Storage Methods

Dried storage is not the only way you'll be keeping your herbs, as you may choose to keep them in preparations and solvents too:

- Water-based preparations consist mainly of water, and teas are an example of this. These are only good for about 24 hours due to the microorganisms in the water.

- Oil-based preparations last much longer, and you can expect a lifespan of up to 3 years.

- Alcohol-based preparation can last 3–5 years, as the alcohol slows down the degradation of the organic material. Yet, while it may last longer, it would be best to use these within 2 years after preparation.

- You can also use vinegar as a preparation solvent; the high acidity of the vinegar will prohibit the growth of bacteria, extending the lifespan of the preparation.

Harvesting or growing herbs, treating them in the correct manner, and storing them appropriately in your apothecary are all tasks to be done with passion and love for the alternative approach to healing. It is a process that reminds us of the way ancient civilizations used herbal remedies coupled with a spiritual element to achieve healing. I am not saying that you have to apply the same practices as the shamans of Northern America or the sangomas in Africa, but spending time in such great awareness of nature surely impacts us on a deeper level than merely the physical. That said, are you ready to discover how you can use your herbal remedies to bring forth healing?

Message from the Author

I am reaching out with immense gratitude for your support in reading this book. Your enthusiasm and feedback mean the world to me, and I would be honored if you could take a moment to share your thoughts.

Your reviews not only provide valuable insights for potential readers but also contribute to the book's visibility. Whether it's a brief comment on what resonated with you or a detailed reflection on the value you gained from the content, every review helps build a community of readers and spread the message of natural medicine.

To leave a review, scan one of the QR codes with your smartphone camera to be taken to the review page.

US   **UK**

Your honest opinions make a significant impact, and I am genuinely excited to hear what you think. Thank you for being a crucial part of this Naturopathic journey.

Warm regards,

Stephen H Sharp

Chapter 5:

Herbal Remedies for Every Ailment

Probably the greatest obstacle keeping people from transitioning from pharmaceuticals to using herbal medicine is the widespread lack of knowledge in this regard. The sad reality is that not only has our generation bought so deeply into the Rockefeller vision, but so have those generations who preceded us. As a result, we've lost a wealth of knowledge along the way.

List of Herbal Remedies

Fortunately, while this knowledge may not be as widely known as it used to be, it didn't disappear entirely. The task to gather all the information we can get and pass it on to the next generation is our responsibility though. Therefore, I am sharing the recipes of as many herbal remedies for treating a wide range of ailments as I can fit into this book. Some of the remedies require the mere application of a single ingredient, while others would need to be prepared.

Acid Reflux (Stomach Acid)

At some time in our lives, we all experience the discomfort of heartburn. However, if this is happening to you twice or more per week, what you are experiencing is most likely *gastroesophageal reflux disease* (GERD). Excess weight, unhealthy eating habits, eating too fast, persistent high stress levels, and smoking are all contributing factors to GERD and they make the symptoms worse. These symptoms include chest pain and tightness and coughing, while regular exposure to the high level of acidity can be very harmful to your esophagus too.

Treatment

The best approach is to transition to a healthier way of eating. Habits like chewing food slowly and taking care to chew it finely; avoiding spicy food or food high in acidity; and wearing looser clothes will all improve your symptoms. You can also turn to natural remedies for relief.

Several herbs can improve the symptoms of GERD and reduce its severity and how regularly it occurs. Teas and tinctures of slippery elm, licorice, chamomile, and marshmallow can all effectively reduce acidity in the digestive tract to improve your GERD. Discuss your plans with your doctor before switching to natural remedies to treat your GERD as these aids can interfere with your prescription meds.

Acne

Acne develops when the pores in the skin get clogged by oil or dirt or even a combination of the two. Once it is clogged, it easily gets infected by bacteria from our hands, the surfaces we touch, or even the air around us. The bacteria cause the skin to get inflamed, leading to redness and tenderness in the area. Several factors can cause acne, like clothing that restricts movement, genetics, lifestyle, stress levels, and health concerns like polycystic ovarian syndrome (PCOS).

Treatment

To treat this concern, you'll have to reduce the inflammation in the skin and kill the bacteria at the same time to prevent them from spreading and infecting other parts of the skin. There are several oils that you can apply to the infected area to clear up the acne.

Tea tree oil has natural antibacterial and anti-inflammatory properties. Applying tea tree oil to the affected area will kill the bacteria and reduce the inflammation to clear the skin. Tea tree oil can be harsh, so it is best to dilute the tea tree oil by using a carrier oil like coconut oil, which also has antibacterial and anti-inflammatory properties and is less harsh than tea tree oil. You can dilute the two by using 1 part tea tree oil to 20 parts coconut oil. Apply this directly to the acne spots with a clean cotton swab 3 times daily until the acne has cleared (Huizen, 2023).

Addison's Disease

Addison's disease is quite rare and is linked to hormonal dysfunction. It refers to an inability to create and release adrenal hormones like cortisol. There is no cure for Addison's disease but it can be managed. Symptoms of Addison's disease are sweating, nausea, light-headedness, muscle pain, and personality shifts.

Treatment

Due to the immune support properties of ginseng, it is a helpful aid to strengthen the immune system to provide better protection to the body. Other herbs that can be vital in alternative treatment are herbs that contain high levels of antioxidants, like green tea and turmeric.

Furthermore, you can also include milk thistle and echinacea as both herbs will improve the strength of the immune system and provide support to ensure better hormonal balance.

Alcohol-Related Liver Disease

Excessive use of alcohol over an extended period can cause severe damage to the liver. This is due to the high level of toxins alcohol leaves in the body. Once the liver has been damaged beyond a certain point, there is little left to do about the concern. But certain herbal remedies will slow down deterioration and ease the symptoms. There are several liver conditions that fall into this category, including liver cirrhosis. The symptoms of the disease include weight loss, fatigue, vomiting, confusion, and getting a yellow tone to the skin.

Treatment

Milk thistle has a reputation for being a wonderful aid in treating liver-related concerns. It takes care of liver health and has many protective properties in this regard. It is also a strong antioxidant and helps to clear the body of toxins.

You can also use ginseng as it will ease inflammation in the liver. Adding green tea to your intake will slow down deterioration too, while it also eases the symptoms.

Allergies

There are so many causes of allergies and these can create a range of symptoms, from having a runny nose to congestion and even fever. If allergies aren't addressed, they can cause inflammation in the upper respiratory system which can spread even further. While it is always best to avoid the cause of your allergies, it may not always be possible.

Treatment

Honey is a proven remedy that can bring great relief to those suffering from allergies. This benefit of honey is linked to the fact that it is made of pollen, helping the body to cope better with this allergy.

Stinging nettle is a natural antihistamine and can help to treat the symptoms of allergies.

The anti-inflammatory compounds in peppermint oil can reduce the inflammation caused by allergies, relieving the discomfort and allowing the mucus membranes to return to normal.

The microbial agents in eucalyptus contribute to minimizing the impact of allergies, and, therefore, it will be beneficial to add a few drops to your laundry.

Alzheimer's Disease

This cognitive disorder causes severe deterioration of the neurons and the brain cells they are connecting with each other. The outcome is a gradual decline in behavior, memory, and mental capabilities.

Treatment

Aromatherapy—and specifically the potent aromatic components of rosemary, lavender, lemon, and orange essential oils—can improve the symptoms of Alzheimer's disease. When using these oils, it is always important to remember that you add only three to five drops to a quality carrier oil to dilute the power of these oils.

Other herbal remedies include taking ginkgo biloba as a preventative measure, reducing the chances of developing Alzheimer's while also improving the cognitive functioning of those diagnosed with the disease. Herbs containing anti-inflammatory properties are also helpful as they can ease the symptoms (Holland, 2017).

Angioedema

Angioedema refers to a condition that mostly results from an allergic reaction and it causes swelling in the soft tissue underneath the skin. However, it can also be the cause of other more serious medical concerns like Hodgkin's disease or leukemia. There are two types of angioedema: There's (a) *acquired angioedema*, and then there's (b) *hereditary angioedema*, the latter which refers to the kind that tends to recur. At times, the condition can develop within minutes, and other times, it may develop over several hours. It is painful and can also go along with symptoms like nausea and vomiting; swelling around the eyes; and discoloration of the skin on the hands, feet, genitals, and face. The condition can be triggered by a range of substances that may cause an allergic reaction, like dyes, pollen, active ingredients in pharmaceuticals, and certain foods.

Treatment

Several herbal remedies will bring relief to the condition. Devil's claw root can improve inflammation and help skin lesions—that may develop when the reaction worsens—to heal. Another trusted natural remedy to improve inflammation and the symptoms going along with it is licorice root. The latter also contributes by restoring immune function.

Ginkgo biloba contains anti-allergenic and anti-inflammatory properties and will relieve these symptoms. However, take note that some people may show an allergic reaction to ginkgo biloba, in which case, it is better to avoid this herb.

While these herbs will work on the allergic reaction, goldenseal will improve symptoms linked to the gastrointestinal system and bring relief to stomach pain, diarrhea, and vomiting (*Angioedema*, n.d.).

Anxiety

Anxiety is one of the fastest-growing concerns of the modern age we are living in. This is a result of high stress levels caused by financial strains, competitive work environments, challenging living conditions, and more. These conditions cause high levels of cortisol in the blood for prolonged periods, causing a range of concerns, like increased heart rate, high blood pressure, shortness of breath, and tightness in the chest.

Treatment

Ashwagandha contains adaptogens that can regulate your stress response, and, therefore, it is a helpful support when managing anxiety. You can use it in liquid form or as a tincture.

Chamomile tea or even the extract of the plant has been used for ages to bring about a sense of calm and to improve sleeplessness.

The aroma of the lavender plant also soothes the nerves and restores a sense of calm.

Valerian root has been used for ages to improve depression, insomnia, and anxiety. However, it is best avoided during pregnancy or breastfeeding, and it is not suitable for children younger than three.

Asthma

Several substances can trigger an asthma attack. Experiencing such an attack is a severe medical emergency, but there are several steps you can take to prevent asthma from taking over your life.

Treatment

Asthma is often linked to inflammation and as garlic contains anti-inflammatory properties, it can be used as a supportive treatment. You can also use ginger for the same reason.

Athlete's Foot

This medical concern is uncomfortable and can be painful. It is caused by a fungal infection in the skin. Usually, the condition will start between the toes and form an itchy rash. Later on, it can have a burning sensation and become painful. It can even form blisters and develop ulcers.

Treatment

Apply tea tree oil daily to the infected area. The antifungal and antibacterial properties of the oil will improve the condition and relieve the symptoms. Dilute the oil with carrier oil and heat it slightly before application.

Neem oil can also be helpful due to the same properties it shares. Simply massage the oil into the skin.

Backache

Backache can be the result of a range of causes and while these may all impact back health in different manners, the greatest concern to those suffering from backache is to find effective pain relief while minimizing the inflammation that goes along with the condition.

Treatment

Capsaicin, derived from chili peppers, is an effective pain relief, as it depletes the compound that is responsible for conveying pain from the affected area to the central nervous system. While it is effective in reducing pain, you may have to wait a couple of days before experiencing the relief you desire, making capsaicin a more effective alternative to manage chronic backache.

Ginger contains phytochemicals that reduce inflammation and help to relieve pain in muscles and joints caused by it. Another herb that has the same effect is turmeric. The active compounds in turmeric also reduce inflammation, and, as a result, you'll experience relief from backache.

Feverfew may bring faster results and has been trusted for centuries to improve pain associated with headaches, toothaches, and even stomach aches. But, it should be used with consideration, as the herb can cause side effects like canker sores, and it should be avoided completely when pregnant.

Bee Stings

Unless you are allergic to bee stings that cause your body to go into a serious state of anaphylactic shock, bee stings are mostly only severely painful once they happen. Afterward, the symptoms like swelling, itching, and redness around the affected area gradually improve over time. Yet, you may want to ease these symptoms anyway, and the following herbal medicines can provide you with the solutions you seek.

Treatment

Aloe vera is known for its cooling properties and will soothe the skin around the affected area. You can use either aloe vera gel or simply break off a fresh piece of leaf and rub it on the affected area.

In some cases, the area may become inflamed. In this case, lavender offers the healing power you are seeking, as the plant has natural anti-inflammatory properties and will reduce swelling. Dilute a couple of drops of lavender oil in a carrier oil like coconut oil and apply generously to the bee sting.

Insect bites or bee stings can also cause the area to become infected. For this, you can use several herbs to bring relief to the concern. Witch hazel is a natural antiseptic and you can apply it directly onto the bee sting. It also has astringent properties and will bring relief to swelling and pain. Calendula is also antiseptic and can be used to treat minor wounds or insect bites and stings, so you can also apply this directly to the affected area. You can also opt for tea tree oil, which will reduce pain and keep the area disinfected (McDermott & Collins, 2022).

Bloating

Bloating is caused by indigestion resulting from eating food that is more prone to causing gas like spicy foods, cabbage, or beans. It also results from poor eating habits, smoking, bacterial activity in the intestine, and even talking while eating can cause gas. The average person releases gas 12–25 times per day (Egan, n.d.). However, it can be that you are gassier than this or experience a buildup of gas that can be painful, in which case it may be necessary to reach out for an herbal remedy.

Treatment

Fortunately, nature offers us many solutions to address this concern. Peppermint is a trusted and relatively well-known aid to treat bloating, and you can chew on peppermint leaves, have a cup of peppermint tea, or even use peppermint oil.

Other herbal remedies include anise, coriander, turmeric, caraway, and fennel.

Bronchitis

This often starts as a mere allergy or cold, but the infection can soon spread and cause full-on bronchitis. *Bronchitis* refers to inflammation in the smaller airpipes, called the "bronchi." Symptoms linked to bronchitis are excess phlegm, congestion, headaches, and fever.

Treatment

Having a humidifier will bring great relief, as the warm moist air helps to open the airways and to loosen the phlegm. However, you'll enjoy better results if you combine aromatherapy with this treatment option. Essential oils that will bring relief are thyme, eucalyptus, basil, tea tree, and peppermint.

You can also try ginseng extract. This root extract contains anti-inflammatory properties that will help to reduce the spread of bacteria and aid in recovery.

Bruises

Bruises are the body's response to when it is injured. The blue-purplish spots you see on the surface are due to bleeding inside the tissue underneath the skin. These can be sore and unsightly.

Treatment

Arnica oil can help to alleviate the pain of bruising. As it is easily absorbed through the skin, the anti-inflammatory properties easily reach the place where it needs to work.

Bromelain, found in pineapples, also helps to reduce the swelling and bruising of these injuries.

Essential oils like rosemary, frankincense, and lavender will also bring relief.

Burns

Burn wounds, even minor ones, can be very painful, leave scars, and become infected. Burn wounds are defined as either first-, second-, or third-degree burns. First-degree burns are red and painful and cause some swelling and redness. Second-degree burns are more severe and cause blisters. They also create a thicker swelling. Third-degree burns are very serious and the skin is charred or white. These burns are linked to nerve damage and may, therefore, be less painful than the other two degrees. Nevertheless, they are far more serious medical concerns, and it may not be possible to treat the latter type of burns effectively with herbal remedies, mostly because of the high risk of infection that goes along with these burns.

Treatment

Aloe vera is a trusted aid when it comes to treating first- and second-degree burns. The gel soothes the pain and will speed up healing. It will also reduce scarring. Apply the fresh gel twice daily.

While aloe vera will relieve the pain, calendula will protect the wound from getting inflamed due to its anti-inflammatory properties.

Celiac Disease

Celiac disease is the result of prolonged exposure to gluten if you are already gluten intolerant. The symptoms of celiac disease include stomach aches, nausea, and flatulence, and as it impacts the absorption rate of nutrients, you may experience malnutrition.

Treatment

You have to avoid food that contains gluten, to prevent your condition from worsening. However, turmeric will be helpful for improving your state as it will reduce the inflammation in the intestine caused by your condition. Turmeric also soothes the gut area and will improve nutrient uptake.

Chapped Lips

Except for the fact that chapped lips don't look good, they can be quite sore too. What causes chapped lips? Dry and chapped lips are caused by a combination of factors. Sure, they are more common during the winter months as the extreme cold is quite harsh on your lips, but there are additional factors that also play a role. Dehydration; certain medications; irritation from biting or licking your lips; and excessive sun exposure can all make your lips dry to the point where they get chapped. These are the most common causes, but they can also be the result of smoking, vitamin deficiencies, or even exposure to irritants. The latter can mostly be found in makeup, toothpaste, or even commercially-sold moisturizers.

Treatment

The first step would be to limit exposure to any of the mentioned factors that contribute to chapped lips, but there are also several natural aids to improve the state of your lips.

Applying coconut oil to your lips will leave them feeling soothed and hydrated. The oil is also antibacterial and anti-inflammatory and will speed up healing. Rosehip oil is bursting with vitamin E and does wonders for your skin too. Rosehip will even improve the color of your lips as well.

Aloe vera is also very soothing to the skin and will soften your lips by binding flaking cells. The best way to use aloe vera is in its rawest form; just cut a leaf and use some of the gel dripping from the cutting to apply to your lips.

Chicken Pox

At some point in most people's lives, they get into contact with chicken pox. This is mostly during childhood years when schools would see a rise in absenteeism due to the spread of the contagious disease, which is known for its itchy red dots that leave scarring if scratched.

Treatment

Except for the itchiness of the rash, the symptoms of chicken pox are usually not severe and may even be similar to having a cold. Thus, as the main focus is on reducing the itch, you can take an oatmeal bath; just add the uncooked oatmeal to a warm bath. The antibacterial and anti-inflammatory properties of the oatmeal will reduce the itchiness and prevent infection.

Having chamomile tea will improve sores in the mouth, and you can also apply cooled tea to the rash to soothe it.

Chlamydia

Chlamydia is a sexually transmitted disease that can cause abdominal pain, bleeding after intercourse, fever, nausea, vaginal discharge, and painful urination in women. Men may experience testicular swelling, rectal pain, thick, milky discharge from the penis, and a sore throat.

Treatment

Goldenseal is an herbal antibiotic that can support the body to fight off infection. Echinacea will support the immune system to better defend the body, and so will garlic. An additional infection fighter to consider is oregano oil. As always, when you use an essential oil, dilute it using high-quality carrier oil.

Cold Sores

Cold sores are caused by herpes simplex HSV-1 virus. It is a virus that lives in most adults, and, in some, it causes cold sores, while others are merely carriers of the virus. Cold sores don't look good and can impact your confidence, but besides that, they are also sore.

Treatment

Apply aloe vera gel to the cold sores to soothe the skin. Due to its antibacterial properties, it can also improve infection in the skin.

The extract of rhubarb and sage in an ointment will also bring relief. It will reduce the swelling in the area and reduce the pain.

Common Cold

When the first cooler weather of winter arrives, it means the arrival of the season when many people start to show the first cold and flu symptoms. It is the time known for runny noses, congestion, sore throats, teary eyes, and body aches, to name only some of the most uncomfortable cold and flu symptoms. If you don't take care and step in to give your body the protection and fighting power it needs, these symptoms can worsen and lead to even more serious health concerns.

Treatment

Now is the time to increase your intake of echinacea, as this helps to boost the immune system and give your body the fighting power it needs. Increasing your zinc intake will also help your body to defend itself, while garlic can be taken daily to improve your systems but also to keep you from getting a cold in the first place. Increase your liquid intake by having herbal teas infused with lemon, ginger, and honey.

Constipation

Constipation is hardly a medical condition, but if it persists for too long, you will start to feel several symptoms mostly caused by a buildup of toxins. In many cases, constipation is an irregular occurrence, but many people suffer from chronic constipation.

Treatment

The flowers, leaves, and fruits of the cassia plant are used to make senna. *Senna* is a natural laxative that stimulates the digestive tract. You can have senna tea regularly to relieve the issue within hours.

Other teas that will improve constipation are ginger, licorice root, chamomile, dandelion root, and peppermint.

When you take aloe vera orally through smoothies or in tea, it also has a laxative effect.

Coughs

There are wet coughs and dry coughs and all of them can be brought on by a range of causes. Persistent coughing can be exhausting and can put a lot of strain on your body. It can also cause you to lose out on sleep.

Treatment

While you would need to address the underlying cause of your cough, you may seek immediate relief simply to give yourself a break from coughing. Honey is a trusted aid in this regard as it kills bacteria but also has a soothing effect on the throat. Having a teaspoon dissolved in water may just be the perfect drink. You can also add ginger to this cup, as ginger will help to relax the muscles tensed up from all the coughing. Elderberry extract will also bring relief.

Use eucalyptus for aromatherapy to open the airways and ease congestion. Peppermint drops or a cup of peppermint tea will have the same effect.

Croup

Babies are very vulnerable to chest infections, and even while breastmilk can provide them with immune support, this is only a temporary relief. This is when they can develop *croup*, an infection in the airways that will rob babies and parents of much-needed sleep night after night. One of the most vital concerns to address is the bacterial infection it causes in the throat. It results in severe irritation causing persistent coughing.

Treatment

Several herbs will soothe the throat and ease the coughing. Use thyme, goldenseal, yarrow, garlic, rose hip, red clover, or licorice. Giving your baby a mixture of lemon and rose hip three times daily will also help to fight off the infection and bring soothing relief.

Depression

Depression is a serious mental health concern affecting a large part of the population. Stressful lives, urban living, and unhealthy lifestyle choices are all major contributing factors to the increase in depression cases globally. While you can't heal depression with medication, it can improve the symptoms you are experiencing and, here too, herbal remedies can play an important role.

Treatment

Ginseng is known as a helpful aid to combat low energy levels and increase motivation. As these are both concerns linked to depression, adding ginseng to your diet will help to make you feel more energized.

A cup of chamomile tea also serves as a wonderful mood enhancer and can alleviate the symptoms of depression.

Lavender oil is linked to relaxation, and it can reduce anxiety. Use this essential oil in aromatherapy to improve your mood.

Saint-John's-wort is another herbal remedy you should stock up on if you fight off the symptoms of depression. The herb has been linked to mental health for centuries and is even used in prescription medication treating depression (Galan, 2019).

Diabetes

There are several contributing factors to the rapid increase in the positive diagnoses of type 2 diabetes. This is a health concern that can be managed effectively, but it also brings about a range of health concerns.

Treatment

Several herbal remedies will reduce the impact of diabetes on your life, as they are tools that will enable you to manage your condition effectively.

Apple cider vinegar decreases the glycemic levels linked to a carb-filled meal. The best time to take this is to have two tablespoons full of water before breakfast.

You can also lower your blood sugar level by adding cinnamon to a glass of water or a hot drink.

Fenugreek is used to spice up food, and it not only can reduce cholesterol levels, but it can also contribute to diabetes management. If you find the smell of your urine reminds you of maple syrup, then you know that the fenugreek is working.

Diaper Rash

There are a few other things in life that are as sensitive as a baby's bottom. While you may be very regular in changing your baby's diaper to prevent prolonged exposure to a wet nappy, it can still happen that your baby gets a red and painful rash. The most common causes of nappy rash are a change in your baby's diet; stool or urine irritating the skin; or a diaper that just doesn't sit the way it should.

Treatment

The best way to prevent and treat diaper rash is to ensure that your baby's bottom remains dry and clean. Apply coconut oil during nappy changes to provide an antibacterial and moisturizing protective layer onto this sensitive skin. If the rash is severe, you can also wipe your baby's bottom with apple cider vinegar diluted in water. Urine is high in alkaline, and the acid in the vinegar will restore the balance.

Diarrhea

Diarrhea can be caused by bacteria or viruses. In the case that it is a bacterial infection, contamination usually occurs through the food you ate, while viral infection can spread in a range of ways. Eating too much of something or food to which your body is intolerant like gluten intolerance can also cause diarrhea. Besides the fact that it is unpleasant to experience, you are also facing the risk of dehydration if your diarrhea continues for too long. For as long as you have diarrhea, the food in your digestive tract passes through very quickly limiting the time of exposure for nutrient uptake. This is especially a concern in the colon. So not only are you experiencing dehydration, your body also starts to become nutrient deficient.

Treatment

Echinacea drops in a glass of water will hydrate your body and boost the immune system to fight off the bacterial infection to speed up recovery. While your diarrhea persists, you may want to stop your stomach from working, but remember that your body is busy getting rid of toxins and whatever caused the infection. Therefore, ideally, you would want it to run its course and take herbal remedies that will keep you hydrated and that will help your body fight off the infection.

A highly effective recipe to treat diarrhea is to add a teaspoon of red raspberry, two cloves of garlic, two teaspoons of Oregon graperoot, and half a teaspoon of chamomile to two cups of water. Let it steep for about fifteen minutes and drink it while it is hot.

Dizziness

Dizziness, or *vertigo*, is often linked to spending time on the water and getting seasick. However, at times, you may experience similar symptoms even when on dry land. This very unpleasant sensation is caused by a buildup of fluids in the inner ear. While vertigo in itself is not a severe threat to your health, it can be caused by a range of health concerns, such as having a sinus infection or even several other severe medical concerns like a neck injury or stroke.

Treatment

Ginkgo biloba is one of the most trusted treatment options to improve the symptoms of vertigo. Taking ginkgo biloba oil daily will restore your balance and help you feel much better again.

Dry Mouth

Having a dry mouth at times when you are nervous— like meeting the partner of your dreams or standing in front of an audience waiting on you to address them— is pretty normal. But, if this is a lasting concern, it can be a bit of a problem. This condition is the result of an insufficient supply of saliva.

Treatment

You can drink more water or stay away from drinks that only dehydrate you, but the following herbal remedies will also improve your situation.

Aloe vera juice has a moisturizing effect on the mouth, and so does gingerroot.

Sweet pepper, or capsicum, also increases the production of saliva. You can also try marshmallow root.

Dry Skin (Eczema)

Eczema, or *atopic dermatitis*, causes the skin to appear dry and chapped. In certain cases, skin can even change in color. It is itchy and can be sore and very uncomfortable to experience. Eczema can affect the lives of people of all races and genders, and quite a substantial part of the global population struggles with this dry-skin concern. Several factors can contribute to eczema, from exposure to harsh weather conditions to diet and allergies.

Treatment

Due to the antibacterial and antimicrobial properties of aloe vera gel, it is soothing and can prevent infections in chapped skin. The natural gel also speeds up wound healing and gives the immune system a boost. You can use the fresh gel from leaf cuttings and apply it directly to the skin.

Apply coconut oil to moisturize the skin and soften the surface. Coconut oil will also form a protective layer on top of the skin to prevent inflammation. You can add a few drops of tea tree oil to the coconut oil as this, too, speeds up healing. Remember to always dilute tea tree oil, otherwise it will dry out and burn the skin.

Earache

Earache may be extremely sore and cause you a great deal of discomfort but it is seldom the result of a severe health concern. Nevertheless, as it is such an unpleasant experience, you will want to resolve it as soon as you start to notice something is off in your ear.

Treatment

Eating raw garlic will reduce the pain as garlic contains lots of *allicin*, which is the active ingredient that fights off bacteria. Another way to combat the bacterial infection is to heat up tea tree oil just slightly and add a few drops to the ear. First, dilute the tea tree oil with a carrier oil like sweet almond oil before applying it to the affected area.

Ginger juice is a helpful aid to relieve the pain that goes along with ear infections. Apply the juice gently around the ear canal. While you will experience relief from pain, it will also help to fight off the inflammation.

Endometriosis

Endometriosis refers to tissue growth taking place on the outside of the reproductive organs. It can affect the ovaries, uterus, fallopian tubes, and surrounding tissue. There is no cure for endometriosis, and, even after medical intervention, it will most likely continue returning. However, you can manage your condition very effectively.

Treatment

Curcumin, the active ingredient in turmeric, is an effective anti-inflammatory aid and will also help to relieve the pain that goes along with endometriosis. It can also help to lower the production of estradiol, linked to endometriosis. Curcumin will also help to minimize tissue migration taking place in the uterus.

Having a cup of chamomile tea can reduce the pain and symptoms linked to the concern, and so can peppermint and ginger. These can all be taken in the form of tea.

However, you can also use lavender, cinnamon, and rose oils diluted in almond oil as an effective aromatherapy treatment to reduce the pain you experience.

Fatigue

Everyone feels tired from time to time, especially if you've been working hard all day, but *chronic fatigue syndrome* (CFS) is somewhat different. It is a state that can become so severe that you can't even take care of your daily tasks. Regardless of whether you are resting in between, you just don't get better. Other symptoms that go along with CFS are muscle and joint pains; mood changes; chills; headaches; and a sore throat or swollen glands. Certain infections may trigger CFS, as it is considered to be the result of an immune system response.

Treatment

Due to its energy-boosting properties, ginseng plays an important role in the treatment of CFS. This delivers the best results if used in combination with echinacea. With CFS being the result of an immune system reaction, these two immune-boosting herbs speed up recovery. In addition, the echinacea will also reduce inflammation in the muscles and joints, reducing the pain you are feeling. Furthermore, you can also rely on peppermint, jasmine, and rosemary essential oils to help minimize the increased stress you experience in this state.

Fibromyalgia

This medical concern, an autoimmune disease, can take over your entire life. It goes along with symptoms like pain in the joints, muscles, and ligaments; fatigue; and body tenderness. It is a disease linked to the nervous system, and, therefore, it can affect the entire body.

Treatment

The number one concern is to bring about pain relief. Here, capsaicin can be a helpful aid. The best way to apply capsaicin is in the form of a cream rubbed into the most severely affected areas.

Fingernail Infections

Various organisms can find a spot underneath your toenails and start to multiply. Regardless of whether it is fungi, bacteria, or even mold, you would want this condition to clear up as quickly as possible. The toenail will discolor and may even fall off if the condition worsens.

Treatment

Soak your feet regularly in a strong blend of plain black tea. The tea contains high levels of tannins that dry out the skin and this kills the bacteria. The tannins also close the pores in the skin to prevent a repeat infection.

Essential oils that you can also apply to the affected area are lemongrass, tea tree, oregano, thyme, cinnamon, or lavender. You have to always dilute essential oils in carrier oil as essential oils are so concentrated.

Flu

Influenza, or the *flu*, is caused by a viral infection. While the flu is quite a common medical concern and is a highly contagious illness that usually affects many—especially during the winter season—it can become a health risk if not taken care of properly. The flu causes fever, headaches, pain, and respiratory concerns. It can also lead to diarrhea and nausea at times.

Treatment

Echinacea will help to boost your immune system to better fight off the threat of the flu, while it also has several properties to help your body defend itself against viral infection. Licorice root will also make a helpful contribution to improving immune defense, and it reduces the rate of virus uptake in the cells.

Ginseng can improve the health of, specifically, the upper respiratory system, while elderberry extract can bring overall relief to all the symptoms you may experience.

Fungal Infections

Fungal infections can be easy to get and are not considered a serious health concern. It can be unpleasant to experience though, as these infections can be sensitive or even painful, itchy, and unsightly. Fortunately, there are many herbal remedies to treat this concern effectively.

Treatment

Tea tree oil diluted into a carrier oil, or apple cider vinegar diluted with water, can be applied to the area, as these aids are high in antifungal properties and can reduce the spread of the fungus. Plain yogurt contains lots of healthy bacteria that prevent the fungus from spreading and is considered to be one of the best treatment options available to address this concern. You can apply the yogurt directly onto the affected area, leave it on for a while, and then wash it off.

Turmeric is another solution that contains antifungal properties. Mix dried turmeric into carrier oil to make a paste and apply it to the affected area.

Ganglion Cysts

A *ganglion cyst* is a sac that forms on the joints or tendons and is filled with fluid. Ganglion cysts develop mostly on feet, hands, fingers, and wrists but aren't limited to only these areas. While they are completely harmless, it can be that you just don't like the appearance of these sacs bulging through your skin, or, in some cases, they can prevent proper movement simply because they are in the way. At times, you may also experience mild pain caused by a ganglion cyst.

Treatment

Frankincense essential oil is analgesic and anti-inflammatory and will reduce the pain you may experience. In addition to that, it also speeds up healing. You can rub a few drops of the essential oil directly onto the affected joint twice daily.

Another pain-relieving essential oil you can use is lemongrass. Dilute the lemongrass essential oil with coconut oil and apply it to the affected area. After 20 minutes, you should wash it off.

You can also rub castor oil onto the affected joint before covering the area with a bandage to keep it warm. After half an hour, remove the bandage and wash off the castor oil. The oil contains ricinoleic acid, which has anti-inflammatory properties.

Gallstones

Gallstones will cause symptoms like nausea and vomiting, and pain in the right abdominal side and back. While larger gallstones need to be surgically removed, it is possible to get rid of smaller stones by using herbal remedies.

Treatment

A tea made of 10 grams of dried dandelion and steeped for 10 minutes in 150 milliliters of water will help to clear the liver, improve digestion, rid the body of gallstones, and get bile flowing again. Take this tea three times a day (Reis, 2022). Milk thistle will have the same effect. Use 1 teaspoon of crushed milk thistle in 1 cup of water. Allow it to sit for 15 minutes before straining the fruit and having the water 3–4 times per day.

Turmeric will reduce any inflammation and pain linked to gallstones. Even if you had surgery to remove these stones, turmeric will speed up cell regeneration and recovery.

Genital Herpes

Herpes is a sexually transmitted disease, but it can also affect other areas of the body as there are several types of herpes viruses. There is no known cure for herpes, but you can take several remedies to improve the symptoms you experience. These are symptoms that vary from pain and irritation to discomfort.

Treatment

Aloe vera will soothe the skin of the affected area. It can also speed up recovery of the herpes lesions. Diluted tea tree oil's antiviral properties will also bring relief, and so will witch hazel due to its antiviral properties.

Chamomile tea can bring about soothing from the inside, but you can also apply diluted chamomile essential oil to the affected area. Other essential oils you can use are ginger, thyme, and lavender oil.

Lemon balm doesn't need a carrier oil and is another known aid to suppress the outbreak and the risk of transmission of herpes.

Glandular Fever

The specific virus causing glandular fever is called the Epstein-Barr virus. The virus is related to the herpes family and causes symptoms like headaches, fever, sore throat, spleen enlargement, and severe exhaustion. It is a common virus found in most adults. However, the number of serious infections is minimal compared to how common the virus is.

Treatment

As it is a viral infection, you'll need to reach for those herbs with antiviral properties. Here, echinacea is at the top of the list, but you can also use olive leaf and Saint-John's-wort. To address the fatigue linked to the medical concern, you can use ginseng or Rhodiola.

Gout

Gout is widely known as a painful inflammation in the joints. It is a type of arthritis that also goes along with swelling of the joints. It can also affect all parts of the body, and you can even experience gout in your ears. The concern is worsened by the consumption of alcohol, stress, and eating food high in protein—specifically red meat—and it is also linked to genetics.

Treatment

The most prominent concern to address is inflammation as this will also improve the level of pain you may experience. Gingerroot steeped in boiling water and left to cool will help a great deal. Other steps you can take are to drink more water; be more active; change your eating habits by reducing your sugar and alcohol intake; and drink apple cider vinegar water. While apple cider vinegar is acidic, it helps to reduce the pain and inflammation caused by gout.

Gum Disease (Gingivitis)

Several factors can contribute to gum disease or gingivitis. At times, it can be caused by poor dental hygiene, but it can also be the result of abrasive brushing, medication, a poor diet, nutrient deficiencies, and smoking. Once the gums get infected, it becomes red and swollen and can start to bleed. It is also prone to pull away from the tooth surface, creating a pocket for bacteria to fester and worsen the problem.

Treatment

Green tea helps to reduce inflammation as it is high in antioxidants. It is especially helpful to reduce inflammation in the mouth, while the polyphenols it contains stop the growth and spread of bacteria.

Another way to clamp down on the inflammation is with turmeric paste. This root is high in antimicrobial agents and rich in antioxidants to fight off inflammation.

Rinsing with a sage mouthwash will also prevent the spread of bacteria, and it combats plaque. Allow two tablespoons of dried sage to simmer in a cup of water for ten minutes. Strain the rinse and let it cool down. Rinse your mouth twice daily for about half a minute.

Hair Loss

Several factors can contribute to excessive hair loss: Stress, hormones, sickness, medication, or exposure to natural elements can all have an impact on your hair. While it is normal to lose some hair daily, you'll need to take certain steps if the problem gets too severe.

Treatment

Add licorice root to your hair routine. The plant extract will open pores and add strength to your hair. It can also improve a dry scalp.

Adding onion juice to your scalp twice weekly will improve circulation and encourage growth.

Rosemary oil, jojoba oil, and aloe vera are all also helpful aids.

Hand, Foot, and Mouth Disease

This is a viral infection with a high contagion rate. It is a common medical concern amongst younger children and causes painful sores on hands, feet, and mouths. However, in more severe cases, you can also get lesions on the buttocks, elbows, and legs. The incubation period for the virus is about six days during which there will be no symptoms, but then the blisters will start to show. The virus spreads through fluid from the nose and throat, while the blisters can also spread the virus.

Treatment

Coconut oil will help the sores to heal and you can also drink gingerroot tea, as this too speeds up healing.

Rooibos tea is an anti-inflammatory tea, and it helps the body to fight the virus, while echinacea and elderberry will support the immune system to improve the body's defense.

Use the aroma of lavender essential oil to ease pain and bring about a night of peaceful sleep.

Hangover

The term *hangover* and its causes hardly need any explanation; in simple terms, it refers to a state after excessive drinking causes a buildup of toxins in the body. This is a state worsened by indulging in cheap alcohol, containing higher levels of toxins. Symptoms include severe headaches, nausea, and fatigue, and it even lowers your immunity.

Treatment

Mint in the form of tea will help to improve nausea, while turmeric will improve the inflammation and pain caused by being in such a state. Turmeric will also speed up cell recovery and repair.

Rosemary will improve any digestive concerns caused by the hangover and will boost your energy levels. Chamomile will also improve digestion, while fennel can take care of nausea.

Parsley, being a diuretic, helps the body to clear itself of these toxins.

Head Lice

Head lice can be a common concern in elementary school as it spreads easily between friends playing in the playground. Lice are small parasites requiring only a minimal amount of blood to survive. They'll live off their host for 24–48 hours and only live on the scalps of humans.

Getting rid of head lice is a challenge as they are so hard to see with the eye. They are light in color and very small, and while they are alive, they can lay thousands of eggs. When you are clearing hair of lice, it is important to remove the nits too. These are even harder to spot and have to be removed by hand, using a fine comb.

Treatment

Tea tree oil contains active ingredients that can kill these lice. You can either mix in a few drops of tea tree oil into shampoo to wash your child's hair or dilute it into a carrier oil to rub into their hair and scalp.

The application of neem oil is much the same in that it disrupts the lice's life cycle and serves as a helpful aid. You can also use lavender oil as it may kill the lice, but doesn't affect the nits. You have to repeat these treatments a number of times. Always remove the dead lice and nits with a fine comb until you can't find any in their hair any longer.

Hemorrhoids

Hemorrhoids are painful and can rob you from enjoying your life. While it is a medical concern you can manage effectively, it may be that, in severe cases, you'll have to get them surgically removed. Hemorrhoids are not a disease but rather a condition. It is part of your body, but it got displaced due to several causes, like childbirth, for example. Except for being painful, hemorrhoids can also be itchy.

Treatment

By applying diluted apple cider vinegar, you'll enjoy pain relief and the itching will lessen. However, refrain from applying apple cider vinegar too often as it may irritate the already sensitive skin. Tea tree oil should be diluted as you may burn the specific area if not, but it can be beneficial by reducing inflammation and swelling, which will also improve the itching and pain.

Hiatal Hernia

Hernias can happen in several parts of the body, but *hiatal hernias* are probably the most common form of hernias. These hernias occur when the stomach presses through the hiatus. The *hiatus* is part of the digestive system linked to the esophagus. These hernias are often the result of an unhealthy lifestyle while they can also occur from excessive pressure on the abdominal muscles. The symptoms include heartburn; difficulty swallowing; feeling bloated or full after eating; and even shortness of breath.

Treatment

Drink apple cider vinegar. Most people would avoid apple cider vinegar when they are already dealing with excessive acid in their digestive system. What few people know is that when you drink this vinegar diluted in water, it creates an alkaline environment and brings relief to heartburn.

This is also a condition that often causes gastric inflammation; for this, you can take half a teaspoon of cinnamon in a glass of water. Cinnamon will also relieve heartburn. A cup of chamomile tea steeped for five minutes will also relieve heartburn, improve gastric inflammation, and lower the acidity in the lower parts of the gastric system.

High Cholesterol

High levels of what is widely known as "bad cholesterol" can become a life-threatening risk. While swapping out your current diet and lifestyle choices for healthier alternatives will already bring about improvement, there are also several other herbal remedies you can try to see an improvement in this regard.

Treatment

Garlic—either raw or in cooked form—reduces blood pressure and improves cholesterol levels. As a result, it slows down the process of atherosclerosis.

As high cholesterol levels put unhealthy high pressure on the heart, it is best to take better care of your heart health. For this, you can use hawthorn. The berries, flowers, and leaves of this plant have been trusted for centuries to improve cardiac health. Do note that hawthorn may interact with prescription medication, so it is best to get a professional opinion from your herbalist before using the herb.

Incontinence

While incontinence is not a serious medical concern, it does take away some quality of life. It is a concern that impacts your social life and confidence tremendously. Several contributing factors cause this inability to properly manage bowel movement, but it is often due to pregnancy and childbirth; chronic bladder infections; or injury.

Treatment

To treat incontinence, you'll likely need a blend of herbs that will include horsetail, nettle, Saint-John's-wort, and buchu. These herbs will also bring relief in the sense that they reduce urinary tract infections, diarrhea, and constipation caused by incontinence.

Indigestion

Indigestion can take on many forms, from nausea and heartburn to bloating, hiccupping, belching, and farting. As the digestive tract is quite long, the cause of indigestion can occur in any place along the system, meaning somewhere in the stomach, gallbladder, bowel, liver, or pancreas. Many factors can lead to indigestion, from the food you eat to your eating habits, a lack of healthy microbes in your digestive tract, and even bacterial activity.

Treatment

There are several herbal remedies you can rely on to improve your indigestion depending on the specific symptoms you are experiencing. If you are mostly struggling with nausea, ginger will be a helpful aid. You can add fresh ginger to your food or enjoy a cup of hot ginger tea.

To relieve bloating, flatulence, and belching, you can use basil. Add the herb to your food. The linoleic acid found in basil contains many anti-inflammatory properties that will relieve the cause of your indigestion.

Drinking a cup of licorice root tea a couple of times a day will also improve digestive concerns. Just add one to two teaspoons of the dried root powder to a cup of hot water.

Insomnia

Your holistic wellness depends on getting enough sleep. While one night of poor sleep won't have any lasting effect, struggling several nights in a row will surely leave you feeling irritable, lacking focus, being moody, and suffering from several other physical concerns. Several factors can contribute to insomnia, and it is best to identify what it is that is keeping you from getting your well-deserved rest and then address that concern. You can also try any of several herbal aids to make falling asleep easier for you.

Treatment

Valerian root is a known aid to improve anxiety, the symptoms of menopause, and depression, and it will help you to enter a state of relaxation and mental calm before bedtime. The aroma of lavender oil is also relaxing and induces sleep, so smelling lavender oil may help you to put an end to your insomnia. You can also opt to have a cup of passionflower tea or chamomile tea about an hour before you head off to bed.

Irritable Bowel Syndrome

Irritable bowel syndrome (IBS) can have an impact on every part of the digestive tract and causes symptoms like diarrhea, spasms, bloating, and constipation. While this is not considered to be a serious health concern, it can be the cause of a great deal of discomfort and pain.

Treatment

Peppermint oil and ginger will ease the buildup of gas and reduce the pain that causes. Peppermint oil also helps to relax the gut muscles and reduce painful spasms. Ginger contains antibacterial agents and will support gut health, but it also includes sedative properties that will reduce pain.

Aloe vera will bring relief to diarrhea and constipation while also improving inflammation in the digestive tract.

Kidney Infection

Sustaining kidney health is essential to maintain overall wellness. While kidney failures may initially appear to be less severe, they can quickly become a matter of great concern as kidney infections that go untreated can develop into kidney failure. This kind of infection is caused by bacteria that enter the kidneys through the urinary tract from the bladder. The symptoms linked to kidney infections are a pain in the lower back and abdomen; nausea and vomiting; smelly urine; and fever.

Treatment

Due to the anti-inflammatory compounds in garlic, it is a wonderful aid to treat this kind of infection. It is also a diuretic and will help the kidney to rid itself of toxins. Garlic is also antifungal and antibacterial, helping the body fight this infection.

You can also use turmeric to bring relief to kidney infection as it will improve cell repair and stop the bad microbes from growing, effectively slowing down the infection. Both garlic and turmeric can be added to your food. Two to three garlic cloves daily would suffice. For the very same reasons, you can also use ginger, while cranberry juice will slow down the growth of bacteria in the bladder and the walls of the urinary tract.

Kidney Stones

Kidney stones develop when there are too high concentrations of toxins in the kidneys coupled with dehydration and urinary tract infections. The condition causes severe pain in the lower back and abdomen and will create a constant urge to urinate. You may also find blood in your urine, feel nauseous, and vomit, coupled with chills and fever.

Treatment

Dissolve apple cider vinegar in a glass of water as this will help to dissolve the kidney stones. It also alkalizes the blood and urine which will make it easier for the body to get rid of the stones.

Dandelion root tea made of ground root powder or even tea made from steeping the flowers of the plant in boiling water will help to cleanse the kidneys by stimulating bile production that helps to rid the body of these toxins.

Olive oil helps kidney stones to pass easier through the bladder, and combining that with diluted lemon juice helps to slow down the process of stone formation. Then, you can also use basil, a diuretic for detoxing the body while also supporting kidney function.

Loss of Libido

There are many reasons why you may experience a loss of libido, from health concerns to being under severe stress. The lack of libido doesn't pose any health threats, but it can also be an indication of certain underlying health concerns that may be more severe. However, it can put a strain on your relationship and impact your life.

Treatment

Saffron may be expensive, but it is a wonderful aphrodisiac as well as an antidepressant. The use of the herb is linked with an increase in sex drive—ginkgo biloba can also do the same. Ginseng is another aid that will increase sexual desire and can be taken to resolve this concern.

Lupus

Lupus is an autoimmune disease that occurs when the body's immune system is attacking itself. The condition can't be cured, but it can be managed and there are several herbal remedies you can use to improve the symptoms. These symptoms include constant inflammation in any healthy tissue from joints and muscles to lungs and kidneys.

Treatment

As one of the most concerning symptoms is persistent inflammation, you'll have to include herbs that have anti-inflammatory properties. Turmeric and ginger are great options. These herbs help to minimize inflammation and reduce pain.

Apple cider vinegar can replenish the lack of hydrochloric acid often found in those who suffer from lupus. The natural aid increases the production of the necessary acid and it also serves as a detoxifying agent for the body.

A flare-up is mostly linked to high-stress situations, and here, tulsi, or holy basil, will be helpful for managing your stress levels more effectively.

Then, you can also consider adding coconut oil to your diet, as it supports immune balance. Simply add a teaspoon of this oil to any hot drink.

Lyme Disease

Lyme disease is caused by a bacterial infection that can occur from tick bites. If you are a person who loves to spend time outdoors, you'll know that there are certain times of the year when ticks are more commonly found in the wild, and it is easy to get one stuck on your clothes and to carry it home. Not all tick bites will result in Lyme disease, but if you are bitten, you are at risk of getting sick. Lyme disease causes severe headaches and body aches; fever; rash; fatigue; and swollen lymph nodes. If it goes untreated and gets worse, Lyme's disease can develop into *Bell's palsy*, which is a partial paralysis of the face.

Treatment

A popular alternative treatment to manage the symptoms of Lyme disease is to rely on aromatherapy. The most effective essential oils are cinnamon bark, wintergreen, citronella, oregano, and clove-bud oil.

Garlic can serve as a preventative measure as, due to its antibacterial properties, it appears that those who include garlic in their diet tend to get bitten by ticks less often.

Herbs that can help to fight off the bacteria are cat's claw, sweet wormwood, and black walnut.

Measles

Measles is a contagious disease that often spreads among children. It is a viral infection that causes fever; headaches and body aches; a rash; and fatigue. While it is not necessarily a serious health concern, it is best to get started treating the condition as soon as possible.

Treatment

Margosa leaves contain several antiseptic and antiviral properties that fight the viral infection while also relieving the itching from the rash. You can add these leaves to the tub and take a bath for about 20 minutes in it.

A blend of turmeric and tamarind seeds is also helpful to fight the sickness, and you should take about 350 grams of this powder daily. Licorice root is also an effective cure for measles. Add about a teaspoon of the powder mixed with honey daily.

Menopause

Menopause is one of the many hormonal changes that women go through in their life span. It can start around their mid-40s and will last for several years. It is a period known for feeling emotional, having hot flushes, and excessive sweating, to name only a few symptoms. While menopause is a stage of life and not a medical concern, it is unpleasant to experience and can be a challenging time to go through for many women. But there is relief available.

Treatment

Black cohosh may not be available across the globe, but it is in North America and is a helpful aid to improve the impact of hot flushes.

When it comes to improving your mood, you can use ginseng to give you an emotional boost.

Migraine

A migraine is so much more than a heavy headache. *Migraines* bring about a throbbing pain that causes nausea, and they can put you in bed for a day or two. As migraines affect such a large part of the global population, there are many over-the-counter options you can choose to use. But long before these were ever available, people settled for herbal remedies to relieve their pain.

Treatment

Feverfew has been used for centuries to improve inflammation and pain, including the pain caused by headaches and migraines. You can make tea from the dried leaves. While there are a few minor side effects to using feverfew like bloating and nausea, these are minimal compared to the many adverse side effects you'll find in conventional medication.

Valerian root is another option you can try. This root works wonders to reduce pain, and as it has such a strong relaxing effect, it will help you fall asleep too.

Coriander seeds are another herbal remedy linked to treating migraines. Chew the seeds, add them to your food, or let them steep in hot water to make a cup of coriander tea.

Rosemary oil improves joint pain and works effectively to calm your mind and lift your migraine. Dilute the oil in a quality carrier oil like coconut oil and apply it to the affected areas; or, you can use the oil for aromatherapy. Alternatively, you can also take rosemary oil capsules to put an end to your pain.

Motor Neuron Disease

Motor neuron disease (MND) is usually diagnosed in more mature adults. This medical concern causes gradual overall deterioration until the body gives in entirely. Symptoms include paralysis, loss of speech, trouble breathing, weight loss, drooling, gagging, and the list continues.

Treatment

No treatment will cure MND, but you can rely on several herbal remedies to improve your condition. Herbal bitters—dandelion, goldenseal, milk thistle, peppermint, or chamomile—will increase appetite and hunger. These herbs also encourage the release of hydrochloric acid in the stomach.

Medical marijuana improves anxiety and stress from dealing with such a diagnosis, but it also creates a protective layer around the neurons that contributes to pain relief.

Barberry and goldenseal contain berberine, a salt that slows down the process of deterioration of the neurons. So, include either of these herbal aids in your treatment plan.

Mouth Ulcer

Constipation, high acidity levels, vitamin deficiencies, and hormonal changes can all be contributing factors to mouth ulcers forming on the insides of your cheeks, tongue, the floor of your mouth, and even on your lips. These can be painful, cause discomfort, and make you feel self-conscious. The tendency to develop mouth ulcers seems to be hereditary, and it also appears that women are more likely to develop them than men (*7 Superb Home Remedies*, 2018).

Treatment

Honey is not only tasty, but it works wonders, too, to improve your mouth ulcers. It is antibacterial and helps to retain moisture in the skin to prevent it from drying out any further.

You can also opt to swirl aloe vera juice in your mouth. As aloe vera contains many anti-inflammatory properties, it is a wonderful treatment for mouth ulcers and even stomach ulcers too.

You can also apply coconut oil as this too will stop inflammation, prevent any bacterial spread, and speed up healing.

Multiple Sclerosis

Multiple sclerosis (MS) impacts the entire nervous system and causes symptoms like poor vision, fading memory, weakness in the muscles, and difficulty maintaining coordination and balance. These symptoms get more severe as the condition progresses. As there is no cure for MS, the best approach to this concern is to manage your symptoms as best you can.

Treatment

Ginkgo biloba will improve brain functioning and memory. It can also improve focus and even reduce vertigo that may result from MS. It will also improve fatigue.

Ashwagandha roots, berries, and extracts can improve chronic pain, inflammation, stress, fatigue, and anxiety.

Myrrh is often used in aromatherapy, but it can also improve inflammation and circulation, as it is an antiseptic.

Catnip can bring pain relief and certain parts of the plant contain anti-inflammatory properties. Chamomile will also aid in sleep, improve skin conditions related to MS, and even resolve an upset stomach.

Muscle Cramps

Cramps would hardly constitute a serious health concern, but it is painful and an indication of the body experiencing a deficiency or being under stress. While you'll have to include food sources high in potassium and magnesium in your diet—as a lack of either mineral often results in painful cramps—there are also several herbal remedies you can take to alleviate your concern.

Treatment

Black cohosh is a wonderful aid to reduce and even prevent muscle spasms, as it naturally helps muscles to relax.

When muscles are so tense, they often get inflamed. This is where *bromelain*, an enzyme found in pineapples, can be helpful. The anti-inflammatory properties of turmeric will also be helpful.

Chamomile tea increases glycine in the muscles which reduce leg cramps.

Ginger contributes in several ways, but as it is an aid in improving circulation, it will contribute to preventing leg cramps.

Nausea

Nausea is not a medical concern on its own and is usually a symptom of a range of medical concerns. However, persistent nausea reduces your appetite; leaves you feeling terrible; can lead to vomiting; causes loss of fluid and electrolytes; and is simply unpleasant to experience.

Treatment

Ginger is a known aid to improve nausea and is often used by pregnant women and those undergoing chemotherapy. Peppermint is also trusted for the same reasons. You can have a cup of peppermint tea or take some peppermint oil.

Cinnamon is also linked to improving nausea, so you can add it to a cup of tea, improving your symptoms while hydrating and replenishing some electrolytes.

Nose Bleed

Some people are more prone to nosebleeds than others. Causes of nosebleeds vary from being in a hot and dry environment to taking medication or having infections in your upper respiratory system. Normally, a nosebleed doesn't continue bleeding for long, but you would want to stop the bleeding as soon as possible and take the necessary steps to prevent it from recurring.

Treatment

A cold press on the nose will slow down circulation and cause the veins to contract, stopping the bleeding. You can also use cayenne pepper, which will improve the blood flow and take the pressure away from the bleeding area. Take a teaspoon of cayenne pepper in a glass of water and drink it immediately when your nose starts bleeding.

Nettle is especially helpful to treat nosebleeds caused by allergic reactions. Steep fresh nettle leaves in boiling water and allow the brew to cool down. Dip a cotton pad in the nettle tea and apply it to the affected area to stop the bleeding.

Osteoporosis

Osteoporosis is linked to old age and a deficiency in the bones. This can cause pain and make people vulnerable to bone fractures. In cases where fractures occurred, healing may be slowed and this can cause other health concerns. It is also a health concern linked to hormonal changes.

Treatment

Red clover contains components that are very similar to estrogen. Since estrogen helps to protect bone health and strength, red clover is a beneficial aid to improve bone health. An herb that makes a similar contribution is black cohosh. The herb also contains components that closely resemble estrogen and offers bone protection.

Horsetail contains silicon that stimulates bone regeneration and prevents the loss of bone mass. You can take horsetail as a tincture or tea, or use it in the form of an herbal compress.

Parkinson's Disease

There is no cure for Parkinson's disease, and it is mostly the case that family members have to powerlessly stand by as a loved one slowly deteriorates in front of them. While there is no cure, you can manage the symptoms and even slow down deterioration.

Treatment

The main concern is to slow down the oxidative deterioration that takes place in the body due to the stress caused by aging. Several advanced herbal blends contain the necessary active compound to do just that; these will include safflower, walnut, velvet bean, and more. If Parkinson's disease is a medical disorder you are or a loved one is battling, it will be beneficial to call on a professional herbalist to mix up an herbal blend to slow down deterioration and ease the symptoms.

Personality Disorder

Personality disorder (PD) is not only a physical health concern that can benefit from the use of herbal remedies but also several mental health concerns. PD is a complicated mental concern without any one cure that will resolve the challenges you are facing. But, there are several means available to you to better manage your symptoms and to enjoy greater contentment in life.

Treatment

Kava kava is a wonderful herb that improves fatigue, anxiety, and insomnia. All three are often symptoms of those battling PD experience. Once you've taken kava kava, you'll soon start to feel how your emotions settle and become much calmer and more relaxed.

Valerian is another herb that brings similar benefits and has a trusted reputation to improve conditions that involve mental and emotional well-being.

Poison Ivy

A stroll in nature can turn into a nightmare if you get into contact with poison ivy. However, it can also be that the weed has found its way to your garden, and then it will leave you with a nasty painful rash. Just minimal contact with poison ivy can cause blisters on the skin.

Treatment

Baking soda and apple cider vinegar are both ingredients found in most homes, and you can use either mixed with some water to apply to the skin.

Aloe vera's many soothing properties will also calm the skin after being in contact with poison ivy. Due to its anti-inflammatory properties, it will reduce redness and swelling.

Tea tree oil's anti-inflammatory properties will do the same and improve the redness, irritation, and itching of the skin.

Postnatal Depression

After childbirth, many women struggle with postpartum depression. They feel overwhelmed and under pressure as they need to care for their babies but are not in the correct state of mind.

Treatment

Passionflower can be a helpful aid as it improves sleep quality and combats insomnia.

Ashwagandha improves the body's stress response and can make it easier to manage your new life in this challenging time. Skullcap is another herbal remedy that improves stress and anxiety.

Post-Traumatic Stress Disorder

Post-traumatic stress disorder (PTSD) used to be a mental health concern linked to only those who have been in combat or are in service where they are exposed to trauma regularly. However, today we know much more about PTSD and that it affects far more people than what was initially expected. It causes symptoms like anxiety, depression, and insomnia, and those who suffer from PTSD often have to endure horrible flashbacks.

Treatment

It is important to get professional psychological support when dealing with PTSD, but the following herbs will help to ease the physical symptoms you may be experiencing.

Rose has a strong aroma that has sedative and calming properties. When you are feeling overwhelmed, it will help to smell rose essential oils which will help to calm you down. Other helpful essential oils that can be used in aromatherapy are cedarwood, lemon balm, and ylang-ylang.

Oat straw improves nerve health and can contribute to recovery in this regard.

Premenstrual Syndrome

Most women suffer from some kind of pain or discomfort from their menstrual cycle at some point in their lives, but there are those—and there are many—who have it much worse than just normal menstrual pains. Premenstrual syndrome (PMS) refers to symptoms like headaches, bloating, mood swings, breast tenderness, an increase in anxiety, spotty skin, and even greasy hair. Several factors can worsen the state, so it is best to avoid them. Reduce your salt intake; avoid caffeine and alcohol; and eat foods that are high in calcium to lessen the impact of PMS on your life.

Treatment

Evening primrose oil reduces the impact of certain PMS symptoms. It does wonders to relieve breast tenderness and even improves your mood. Other alternative remedies include ginko, chaste berry, ginger, and Saint-John's-wort. When you opt for any natural remedies, it remains important to discuss this with a health care expert as the use of herbs may impact other areas of your health, especially when you use it with conventional medication. For example, Saint-John's-wort can make your birth control less effective.

Psoriasis

Psoriasis is one of those medical concerns that can have an immense impact on your life, self-image, and confidence, even though it may not be serious at all—medically speaking. It doesn't look pretty; it is itchy and flaky; and it can get inflamed. You can manage your symptoms more effectively through your diet, but these herbal remedies will also improve your condition.

Treatment

Apply apple cider vinegar to the affected skin to improve the itchiness. While you can apply this either diluted or full strength, don't use this treatment if the skin is broken or cracked.

Add capsaicin to your diet to reduce the inflammation in the skin caused by psoriasis. It will also reduce the pain you may experience.

Having turmeric quite regularly as part of your diet can reduce the severity and frequency of flare-ups of psoriasis.

Tea tree oil can also help, especially if the scalp is an affected area. All you need to do is to drip a few drops into your shampoo.

Ringworm

Ringworm is not an actual worm but, in fact, a parasite living in the skin, leaving a mark resembling a worm. This causes an itchy and dry area that can easily get inflamed.

Treatment

You can soak the affected area with diluted apple cider vinegar three times daily.

Tea tree oil and the many beneficial properties it has will also treat the fungal infection in the skin effectively. Applying turmeric to the skin will have a similar effect.

Coconut oil will also treat the infection while moisturizing the skin.

Rosacea

Some call it rosy cheeks, but *rosacea* is something that can leave you feeling self-conscious. It is caused by tiny blood vessels right on the surface of the skin, giving the skin a red, or even sometimes purple, tone. When the skin is dry, it can easily get inflamed causing red blotches on the surface of your skin.

Treatment

Lavender has the soothing qualities you need to improve the appearance of rosacea.

Feverfew will prevent blood from pooling in these blood vessels and make it look even worse.

Oatmeal applied to the skin soothes it and reduces redness and itching.

Scabies

Scabies refers to a condition where mites burrow their way into your skin, causing itching and the risk of inflammation. It also causes blisters and red skin.

Treatment

Tea tree oil will stop the itching and can impact scabies, even though it doesn't kill the eggs deep in the skin.

Neem oil can kill the mites and resolve the concern.

Aloe vera will also improve the symptoms of scabies.

Shingles

Shingles are painful, itchy lesions that can appear across the face and body. It occurs when the herpes virus is activated, often due to stress.

Treatment

Several essential oils can be helpful to treat shingles. Try using chamomile, tea tree, and eucalyptus oil; these all have anti-inflammatory properties and will work in the affected areas.

Witch hazel will improve the itching and pain.

Scarlet Fever

History tells a tale of how devastating scarlet fever can be, but today, we've got a much better grip on the sickness. *Scarlet fever* is caused by streptococcal bacteria and mostly affects children between the ages of two and eight. Symptoms include vomiting, small red spots on the skin, swollen lymph nodes, headaches, fever, and a sore throat. It takes about seven days from infection to showing the first symptoms.

Treatment

While raw honey will boost the immune system, you can also add 1 cup of regular honey, 2 cups of apple cider vinegar, and 1 cup of Epsom salt to the bath. Let the child sit in the bath for about 20 minutes to improve the rash. Once dry, add coconut oil to provide a moisturizing antibacterial layer to the skin.

You can also use elderberries in syrup form or as a tincture. The active compounds in elderberries will speed up healing.

Sepsis

Sepsis is a severe medical concern that poses a high risk of mortality. *Sepsis* refers to a state of infection in which your entire body reacts to a bacterial or fungal infection. It can start in the kidneys, spread to the abdomen, and, from there, gradually move to every part of the body. This is a serious medical concern, but, that said, you can use herbal remedies to support the treatment and speed up recovery.

Treatment

Turmeric remains the trusted aid to fight off infection, and it will do the same in this case by reducing swelling and pain. Make a concoction of turmeric and water and drink that daily.

Combine garlic and honey. The anti-inflammatory, antibacterial, and anti-fungal properties coupled with the immune-boosting power of honey will support recovery. Have a teaspoon of minced garlic and honey daily.

Sinusitis

At first, it might have started out as merely a couple of sneezes, but, soon, your allergy has caused such severe irritation in the mucus membranes of your nasal cavity that you are stuck with *sinusitis*. The term refers to inflammation in the hollow spaces in your nose, cheekbones, and forehead which are called the sinuses. Once these areas become inflamed, they can cause swelling. Coupled with an excess of mucus, you'll feel congested and heavy-headed; struggle to breathe; have a fever; struggle to taste anything; and you can also expect to have a headache.

Treatment

The best approach to bring this to an end is to act fast before the inflammation spreads to other areas along your air passages. Start by eliminating any dairy products from your diet, as dairy causes an excess of mucus and will counter all your efforts to relieve your symptoms.

Furthermore, it is important to hydrate as much as possible as this will ease the congestion in your sinuses.

Once the congestion becomes less severe, the inflammation will ease and so will the pain.

You can also steam yourself. Add a few drops of eucalyptus oil to the water to clear up the congestion you have.

Another natural remedy is to increase your intake of bromelain. *Bromelain* is a mixture of various enzymes found in fresh pineapples; it clears up sinusitis and the inflammation causing it.

Stomach Ulcer

Stomach ulcers are open sores on the inner lining of the stomach, and they are often caused by high acidity in the stomach due to diet, unhealthy lifestyle choices, and stress. Certain harsh medications such as aspirin can also irritate the stomach lining, worsening the situation. These open sores are at risk of getting inflamed due to bacterial exposure, and then they can become a much greater health concern. If you are diagnosed with stomach ulcers, it is vital to make serious changes to your lifestyle. In addition to this, you can also rely on several natural remedies to speed up healing.

Treatment

Flavonoids have earned a reputation for being outstanding in treating stomach ulcers. You can find these in a range of fresh fruits and vegetables like berries, legumes, red grapes, broccoli, and apples.

Flavonoids protect the inner lining of the digestive tract and speed up healing.

Honey is sweet and tasty but also a powerful natural remedy loaded with antibacterial properties. It does wonders to speed up the healing of stomach ulcers, and as long as you have no blood sugar concerns, you can include this in hot beverages or on food.

Garlic slows down the growth of bacteria that negatively impacts the state of the stomach lining and worsens stomach ulcers. Add fresh garlic to your meals to slow down the spread of this bacteria.

Cranberry juice is not only excellent for treating urinary tract infections but also stomach ulcers as it, too, reduces the presence and spread of bacteria.

Stress

We all feel the impact of stress, but when it gets out of hand, it can be truly dangerous to your health and well-being. High stress levels are linked to a range of health concerns like heart disease, strokes, high blood pressure, and even stomach ulcers. While you can treat all these symptoms, you would also want to improve the level of stress you experience. It may be that you have to make certain lifestyle changes, make time to relax, and get more exercise. However, several natural remedies will also support your quest to better manage your stress.

Treatment

Sip on a cup of chamomile tea. Chamomile has been trusted for years to improve stress and anxiety. The same is true for passionflower tea, making it another hot beverage you can have to improve your stress levels. The same goes for valerian root, which is often stirred into a cup of hot water to improve depression, anxiety, and insomnia.

Lavender is a wonderful option for aromatherapeutic relief. The smell of lavender is naturally calming and soothing, and it will even help you to fall asleep.

Sunburn

Having fun in the sun can turn into a nightmare when sunburn steps in. Sunburn is painful and causes a great deal of discomfort. It can also leave lasting scars. In severe cases, sunburn can even leave blisters and swelling of the skin.

Treatment

Aloe vera gel will soothe the skin. You can also apply the gel from freshly cut aloe leaves directly onto the affected areas.

Applying witch hazel with cotton gauze and then washing it with water for about 20 minutes will also soothe your skin and reduce the pain. The herb's tannins are anti-inflammatory, thus causing a soothing sensation.

Other remedies include taking a bath in oatmeal and applying coconut oil.

Swollen Glands

The lymphatic system is one of the more complex systems in the body. It consists of ducts, nodes, vessels, and glands. Through this system, the body distributes lymphatic fluids that help to eliminate waste products and to distribute immune cells to where it is needed in the body. Sustaining a healthy lymphatic system requires a healthy lifestyle, enough sleep, and exercise. At times, these glands can become inflamed and swollen, preventing proper lymphatic drainage.

Treatments

Marigold, or *calendula*, is a trusted aid to improve the swelling and inflammation in the lymph nodes. It is high in anti-inflammatory properties and speeds up healing. Coupled with the immune-boosting power of echinacea, you can clear up the inflammation in your lymphatic system in no time.

Also, consider dandelion, as this is a detoxifying agent that helps the body to clear up any pollutants. Other herbs that can clear up swollen glands are wolf's foot, devil's claw, and goldenseal.

Thrush

Thrush is caused when a large number of fungi are present near the vagina. Thrush symptoms include discharge, pain, discomfort, itching, and irritation.

Treatment

Oregano essential oil contains active compounds that will change the formation of the fungi and reduce the symptoms. Dilute three drops into a carrier oil, like sweet almond oil, and apply it to the affected area. Due to the antifungal nature of coconut oil, it too will restrict the growth of the fungi and speed up recovery.

Taking a bath with half a cup of apple cider vinegar will also help to clear the area of the yeast and other harmful microorganisms.

Thrush in Men

A far less known fact is that men also get thrush. It is caused similarly and the symptoms are also much alike to thrush in women. Men may experience burning when urinating, redness, and itchiness of the penis and surrounding areas; discomfort during sex; and an odor.

Treatment

Dilute tea tree oil in olive oil and apply it to the affected area. As the oil contains antibacterial, antiprotozoal, and antifungal properties, it will improve the condition quickly.

Applying apple cider vinegar and coconut oil will also bring relief to men.

Tonsillitis

You are familiar with the symptoms of tonsillitis. A sore throat, pain when you swallow, fever, ear pain, a horse voice, and bad breath are all symptoms of inflammation in the tonsils caused by either a bacterial or a viral infection. Tonsillitis is easy to address with herbal remedies and the key to your success is to act fast. The sooner you notice any symptoms and start treating, the quicker your recovery and the less painful your throat will be. Unless your condition deteriorates, tonsillitis is easy to treat at home.

Treatment

Gargle with salt water as much as you can. The water will soothe the pain and reduce the inflammation in the area.

You can also sip on warm tea with some honey. This, too, will ease your pain while the honey's healing properties work on your inflammation and ensure the healing you are hoping for. Ginger tea is also high in anti-inflammatory properties and will help to speed up healing. In between, suck on licorice lozenges. Licorice contains many anti-inflammatory properties and will also soothe pain. Also, take care to drink enough fluids to remain hydrated as this will also help your body to fight off the inflammation.

Toothache

Toothache is one of the worst pains there is as it goes into the bone and affects your entire head. It can result from tooth decay, trauma, or infected gums.

Treatment

Peppermint tea soothes the pain and the menthol in peppermint serves as an antibacterial aid to improve the condition. Steep 1 teaspoon of dried peppermint leaves in a cup of boiling water for 20 minutes and, once it is cool enough, use it as a mouthwash to swish in your mouth. Cloves have very much the same effect; soak cloves in oil and apply the oil to the tooth.

Thyme is antiseptic and you can also use a mouthwash of a few drops of thyme essential oil in a glass of water.

Tooth Decay

Cavities can largely be prevented by taking proper care of your teeth, but several herbal remedies will help to prevent this dental concern.

Treatment

Oil of oregano kills off any bacteria and keeps your mouth clean and infection free.

Green tea improves the fluoride in your teeth, keeping them stronger for longer. Adding the support of licorice root—to build up dental strength—will help your teeth even further.

Underactive Thyroid

Most people who have an underactive thyroid are unaware of their medical condition. However, while the medical concern is apparently completely harmless, it can cause several other health concerns that can have far more serious outcomes. An underactive thyroid can cause high blood pressure, weight gain, heart disease, and memory loss. It is also linked to Hashimoto's leaky gut, causing several health challenges.

Treatment

One of the properties of *curcumin*, the active ingredient in turmeric, is that it prevents autoimmune diseases and also supports good thyroid health.

Chasteberry is helpful in hormonal management and can support better hormone balance, making it a supportive treatment for Hashimoto's disease.

Urinary Tract Infection

Most urinary tract infections (UTIs) are caused by bacteria. It is a type of infection that is far more common than you might expect. Nevertheless, it causes discomfort, pain, fever, and fatigue. Women are by far more affected by UTIs than men (Hill, 2023). For many, the only solution is to opt for antibiotics, but several herbal remedies will resolve the problem and relieve your symptoms too.

Treatment

Garlic combats all kinds of infection, whether they are from viral, bacterial, or fungal origins. It contains a sulfur compound called *allicin*, which is what holds its healing power. Add garlic to your meals to experience relief.

Cranberries have become such a popular remedy for UTIs that you'll find them in many OTC options too. The berry juice slows down the growth of bacteria and can even prevent UTIs, a factor to consider if you are prone to regular infections.

Green tea is another great way to address this concern due to its antibacterial and anti-inflammatory properties. Other herbal teas that can also be helpful are mint, parsley, and chamomile tea.

Varicose Veins

Varicose veins are small veins that move to the surface as they are under constant pressure. While they affect the appearance of the skin in these areas, they are also sore at times, and you may experience throbbing pain in your legs. They are uncomfortable and can cause cramps and may be itchy. The condition can also cause swelling of the ankles and lower calves.

Treatment

Horse chestnut extraction can improve pain in those areas. A blend of butcher's-broom and sea-pine extract can relieve the swelling. As the skin around these areas is very sensitive, it is vital to dilute any essential oils before application.

Grape-seed extract is another herbal remedy that has proven itself to be a trusted remedy to improve the condition.

Venous Leg Ulcer

Skin ulcers are often wounds that just don't heal. These should be carefully treated, as they expose the body to infection. They are also painful, itchy, and can spread to the surrounding areas. These wounds also often contain bacteria that prevent them from healing, so this should also be addressed as part of the treatment.

Treatment

Comfrey, aloe vera, arnica, calendula, and slippery elm are all helpful herbs that can contribute to healing. These herbs will reduce inflammation and improve circulation in the affected area.

The flowers of calendula can be infused into an ointment and applied to the wound, while aloe vera gel can be applied directly from a freshly cut leaf.

Warts and Verrucas

Warts don't have to be a challenge to remove, especially if you apply early intervention.

Treatment

Apply apple cider vinegar to the area. The high acidity in the vinegar will gradually eat away the infected skin and remove the wart over time. Dilute the apple cider vinegar with water by mixing two parts vinegar to one part water, and then dip a cotton ball into the mixture to apply to the area.

Garlic can also help due to its antimicrobial effects. Crush one clove and mix it with water into a paste. You need to apply the paste to the wart and cover the area with a bandage. You can also use garlic juice and rub it onto the wart.

Whooping

Whooping cough, or *pertussis*, refers to a condition of a contagious bacterial infection in the respiratory tract. It mostly affects children. Symptoms are a slight fever, sneezing, loss of appetite, and a mild cough. The first stage lasts for about two weeks before it gets worse. During the second stage—which can last up to six weeks—there may be vomiting and long and regular coughing spells, the latter which can develop into pneumonia.

Treatment

Echinacea and garlic will boost the immune system to help the body fight the sickness.

Hyssop and anise can reduce the amount of mucus in the infected area.

Catnip, chamomile, and thyme will reduce the spasms in the area and improve congestion.

Tinctures, Infusions, and Tonics

Herbal tinctures are probably the most potent herbal remedy you'll have in your apothecary. They are easy to make, and you would only need a liquid like alcohol or vinegar along with the specific herb you would like to use for the tincture. Essentially, a tincture is a potent extract containing the active components in herbs. Do keep in mind, though, that not all extracts are tinctures.

To make the tincture, you have to soak the herb for several weeks in the liquid of your choice. While alcohol is the preferred choice for many herbalists, you can also use glycerin or vinegar to make tinctures.

Tincture Method

Once you are more experienced in making herbal medicine, you can explore other ways for making tinctures too—for example, through distillation. But, the method I am sharing is very easy to do at home and you don't need any special equipment:

1. Wash all the parts of the herb you are going to use for your tincture and remove any parts that you don't want.

2. Chop or break these parts into chunky bits and place them in an airtight glass jar.

3. Cover the herb parts with alcohol or vinegar. When you are using fresh herbs, the best ratio is 1:1 with the alcohol; for dried herbs, a ratio of 1:4 is better. Seal the jar.

4. Allow the jar to stand for at least 6 weeks. Shaking the jar regularly will help to release the active components into the tincture.

5. If you see that the alcohol level has dropped, add more to the jar to ensure that the herbs remain entirely submerged in alcohol. As the alcohol you'll be using is so harsh, it can cause corrosion in the lid of your jar. Insert a piece of parchment paper inside the lid to prevent this from happening. Never use plastic jars to make tinctures, as the alcohol will eat away the plastic.

6. After 6 weeks, you can open the jar and strain the alcohol to get rid of the herbs. A clean cheesecloth works best here.

7. Place the cheesecloth inside a funnel and strain the tincture into a clean glass bottle. Once the alcohol has stopped dripping into the bottle, you can give the cheesecloth a good squeeze to get as much goodness into your tincture as possible.

8. Pour the tincture back into the glass jar or stopper bottles, seal it properly, and label it clearly. Remember to include your dates on the label.

9. Store in a cool and dark place until you need it.

Application of Tinctures

As tinctures are so potent, a little goes a long way. Use a dropper to drip only a few drops in your mouth, preferably underneath the tongue. Be sure to hold the tincture in your mouth for a couple of seconds before swallowing.

Benefits of Tinctures

Tinctures are a great addition to any apothecary as they have a longer shelf life than most other remedies. They are also very potent, and, therefore, you only need a few drops at a time. They are easy to make and a convenient solution to treat a range of health concerns.

Tips for Making Tinctures at Home

Tinctures are very easy to make, and the only part that may be tricky is sourcing quality alcohol and knowing what strength of alcohol to use. You'll have to adjust your alcohol strength to the type of herb you are using (Kolen, 2017):

- For **dried herbs**, it is best to use **40–50%** alcohol. An effective solution is to opt for 80- to 90-proof vodka. The lower percentage of alcohol is the most effective for extracting water-soluble components in dried herbs.

- For **fresh herbs or herbs that have a high moisture content**, you should use **67.5–70.0%** alcohol. The higher percentage of alcohol effectively extracts the aromatic properties of the plant and your tincture will contain more plant juices and the goodness it carries. The most effective alcohol blend will be to use a 1:1 ratio of 80-proof vodka and 190-proof grain alcohol.

- **Gums and resins** require an even higher alcohol volume. You won't be able to properly extract the essential oils and aromas in the sticky plant material without a strong enough alcohol in your tincture. So, here you need to use **85–95% alcohol**, which will be 190-proof grain alcohol.

I bet your next question is related to where you find grain-proof alcohol. Sourcing this alcohol is not as hard as you may imagine. Visit your local spirits providers; if they don't stock what you are looking for, they are usually willing to place a special order once you explain what you are doing. If this is not the solution for you, you can also source it from any of several online providers (Kolen, 2017).

Nonalcoholic Tinctures

There are many possible reasons why you may not want to include alcohol in your tinctures, and for this, there is also a solution. Glycerin and vinegar are very effective liquids to use in tinctures too. The correct term to use for a tincture with a glycerin base is "glycerite."

Glycerin is a clear liquid with a slightly sweet taste that is a byproduct when fats and oils are broken down. You can buy glycerin at your local health shop or even at pharmacies. It is a natural ingredient and the perfect substitute for alcohol, especially when you are treating your children from your apothecary. The disadvantage of using glycerin when making tinctures is that it doesn't last as long compared to alcohol tinctures; it will remain good for two to three years. It is also not as effective in extracting active ingredients as alcohol is.

Making a Glycerite

You'll need food-grade glycerin, herbs of your choice, boiling water, a clean jar for extraction, and a bottle to store your glycerite:

1. Break or cut the herbs into chunks and fill the jar about halfway with herb bits. Don't compress the herbs into the pot.

2. Pour just enough boiling water over the herbs to moisten them.

3. Fill up the jar to the brim with glycerin.

4. Add the lid to ensure an airtight seal.

5. Allow the jar to stand in a dark but relatively warm spot for about four weeks. Shake it regularly.

6. After four weeks, you can pour the mixture through a strainer layered with cheesecloth to separate the liquid from the herbs.

7. Clearly mark the bottle, including dates, and store it in a dry, dark place.

Making Tinctures From Vinegar

Vinegar is, of course, another option you can use to make potent tinctures that are alcohol-free. When it comes to the effectiveness of vinegar tinctures, you'll enjoy the same benefits that the ones with an alcohol base will give you. It will even take the same time for the active ingredients to get into your bloodstream. The benefits are that it is safe to give to children and can help you to fulfill more purposes. For example, you can use vinegar tincture in salads too. Another way to use these is as the basis for a hot, cold, and flu remedy. The greatest disadvantage is that these tinctures will last a maximum of one year on the shelf. They are also less potent, so you'll have to take larger dosages.

You'll need the dried herbs you are going to use, apple cider vinegar; a glass jar; cheesecloth and funnel; and the bottles you are using for storing your tincture (Jeanroy, 2022b):

1. Break your dried herbs into smaller pieces, and then fill the jar to the top with herbs without compressing it into the jar.

2. Fill the jar with apple cider vinegar and seal it tightly.

3. Place the jar in a cool, dark spot for two weeks. Shake the jar daily to agitate the contents, as this will ensure proper extraction of the active ingredients.

4. After two weeks, you can pour the mixture through cheesecloth and funnel it into a glass stopper bottle.

5. Clearly mark and label the bottle and store it in a cool dark place.

Tincture Storage Tips

There are a few guidelines you need to adhere to if you want to enjoy the longest possible lifespan from your tinctures.

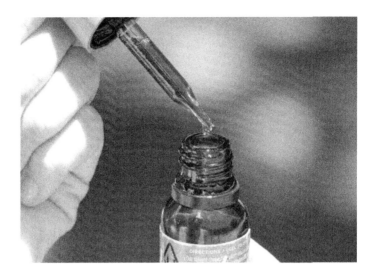

Tinctures with an alcohol basis are usually safe to keep for even longer than five years. Just be sure that you keep them in a cool, dark, and dry spot. Always seal the bottles properly after using them to prevent evaporation.

Glycerites don't have such a long life span and are more prone to getting contaminated with mold. Always check your bottles for any mold growth before use. You'll spot this as white or gray flakes floating on top. Discard the contents immediately when you see mold growing in these bottles. You can follow the same storage guidelines for tinctures made of vinegar.

Making Herbal Antibiotics

Did you know that you can make your own herbal antibiotics? Many herbs are known for their antibacterial, antiviral, and antifungal properties. These are properties they have due to the natural active components present in them.

While it is easy to make herbal antibiotics, it is important to understand that they work in a different way than the antibiotics you'll fill with a prescription. Herbal antibiotics will do the following three things for you:

- It will slow down the growth of bacteria.

- It can even destroy bacteria.

- It will strengthen your immune system to fight off the infection or illness caused by the bacteria.

With this in mind, you need to take herbal antibiotics as soon as you start to feel sick. The longer you wait to address the concern, the longer it will take to see improvement. You also need to be sure that you've correctly prepared the herbal antibiotics. For external wounds, this would mostly be in the form of salves or powders, while for internal infections, you'll use syrup, tinctures, or infusions. You must take the correct dosage based on your body weight and you have to take them consistently, as herbs take longer to work and have a slower effect.

If you don't start to feel better, or even worse, call on a qualified herbal practitioner to be sure that you are using the correct treatment.

The Best Herbs to Use in Antibiotics

The list of herbs containing the properties you would need for an antibiotic is quite extensive, but the following herbs are common choices for this kind of remedy:

- echinacea

- eucalyptus

- garlic

- goldenseal

- hyssop

- red root

- rosemary

- Spilanthes

- usnea

- yarrow

How to Make Herbal Antibiotics

You'll need a glass jar with a lid, a dropper, or any other glass bottle for storage; a strainer; and cheesecloth.

Ingredients:

- ½ cup of fresh rosemary, finely chopped
- ½ cup of fresh garlic cloves chopped
- ½ cup of fresh thyme finely chopped
- ½ cup of fresh ginger chopped
- apple cider vinegar

Method:

1. Allow the garlic to sit for about 10 minutes after chopping it. During this time, it will release more *allicin*, which is an active compound with healing and antibacterial properties.

2. Next, add rosemary, garlic, thyme, and ginger into a glass jar.

3. Top it up with apple cider vinegar.

4. Seal with an airtight seal.

5. Leave the jar in a cool, dark place for about six weeks, but remember to shake it regularly.

6. After six weeks, pour the vinegar through a funnel layered with cheesecloth.

7. Store in a glass or stopper bottle in a cool, dark, dry place.

Dosage:

Take one full dropper on a glass of water three times daily as soon as you start feeling a cold coming on. Continue until the cold or flu has passed (Patiry, n.d.).

Herbal Infusions

Herbal infusions are often referred to as teas, but the accurate term to use to refer to these blends is "tisanes" or "infusions." These blends are usually much stronger than teas and can therefore be risky if taken too often.

Herbal infusions can be used as a drink to address certain internal ailments, for external treatments, in homemade cosmetics, and even as natural insect repellents. Infusions can treat disease but also be enjoyed to support overall wellness, mentally and physically.

Making Herbal Infusions

You'll need a teaspoon of the dried herb you would like to use in your infusion, boiling water, and a clean jar with a lid. Add the herbs and boiling water to the jar and close the lid to prevent any aromas from escaping.

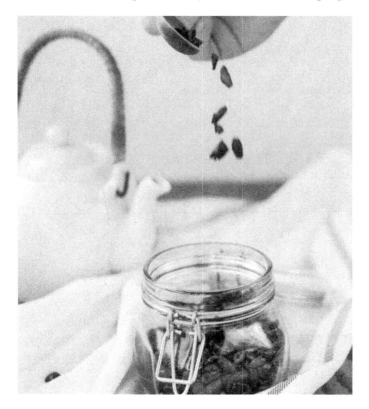

The length of time you'll need to let this steep would depend on what parts of the plant you used. If you've used the bark of the plant, you'll have left the jar for about 8 hours. Bark gives a very potent infusion also known as a "decoction." Leaves should steep for 4 hours, and flowers would need at least 2 hours before you can drink the infusion. Seeds and berries only require 30 minutes of steeping before you can pour the blend through a funnel lined with cheesecloth.

Afterward, you can discard the dried herbs and store the infusion for up to 48 hours if you keep it refrigerated (Jeanroy, 2022b).

The type of herb you'll use would depend on what ailment you want to treat. Every herb has a unique set of healing properties and can treat a range of concerns. The most popular choices for making herbal infusions are the following though (Jeanroy, 2022b):

- **Mint** helps with digestive concerns and improves nausea and vomiting. It also helps to release gas and stomach aches.

- **Lavender** infusion is strong and contains antiseptic properties. Therefore, it is often used to treat external wounds or acne.

- **Echinacea** is a well-known name to combat colds and flu. You will use only the flowers of the plant to make your infusion.

- **Nettle** can bring about pain relief in the joints or pain caused by arthritis. It also improves gout and can relieve eczema.

- **Chamomile** is great to calm the nerves and to combat stress. As it supports sleep, it is often used to treat insomnia. You can also gargle the infusion to treat a sore throat.

- **Sage** infusion boosts memory power and cognitive functioning. The herb contains high levels of antioxidants and is a wonderful aid to fight off inflammation.

- **Thyme** can be gargled to treat mouth and throat infections like sore throats and mouth sores and even to improve bad breath.

- **Oat straw** brings relief to those struggling with cholesterol and can play a helpful role to aid in heart health.

- **Mullein** is a known treatment for lung conditions like asthma. It also fights inflammation.

- **Red clover** contains high levels of vitamins, protein, and phytosterols. The latter has recently started to attract attention as an aid to prevent certain cancers.

The healing power found in herbal medicine and the number of ailments you can treat naturally are truly astounding when you first start to explore the world of alternative medicine. However, herbal medicine is not only a great way to treat health concerns, but also to improve overall health and wellness, both physically and mentally.

Chapter 6:

Herbal Remedies for Mental and

Physical Performance

What I often find is that when people initially show interest in herbal remedies and are keen to make the shift away from pharmaceuticals, they are hoping to at least cut down on some of the prescribed medication they are used to taking. They often believe that while they'll be able to replace some OTC options with more natural alternatives but are unaware of the long list of ailments they'll be able to treat simply by relying on the herbs they have in stock in their apothecary at home. So, if your head is still spinning after learning all you can do with herbs in the previous chapter, it is perfectly normal. But that is not all there is to herbal medicine.

In this chapter, I also wanted to share with you how you can use herbal remedies to improve your overall well-being and to improve your performance on a mental and physical level too. This just proves that herbal remedies aren't only beneficial as a treatment option but also as a preventative and supportive aid.

Herbal Remedies to Improve Sleep Quality

Getting enough sleep is probably one of the most underestimated contributions you can make to sustained health and wellness. Without getting a proper night's rest, you are going to experience physical and mental exhaustion, but there is much more to it. Reduced focus, a limited attention span, increased irritability, poor memory, and feeling moody are some of the other symptoms you may experience too. However, familiarity with all you are exposing yourself to when you are not getting sufficient sleep has never helped anyone suffering from insomnia to enjoy a night of peaceful and revitalizing sleep. Therefore, let's see what can help you out of this predicament.

Lavender

This potent herb with purple flowers is a widely trusted aid for a range of health concerns, of which insomnia is one. Do not take lavender orally as this may cause diarrhea, nausea, and belching. But, as an aromatherapy treatment, lavender has a wonderfully calming effect. As stress is such a major contributing factor toward insomnia, you'll already find it much easier to fall asleep once you've got a stress management regime that works for you.

Taking a warm bath infused with lavender essential oil or just smelling the scent of lavender before bedtime will help you to fall asleep much easier.

Passionflower

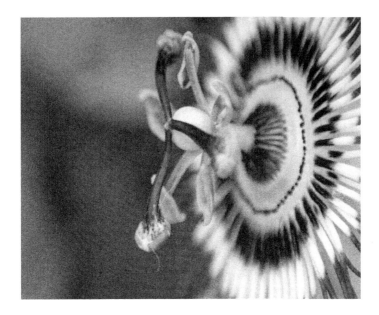

The flowers of the passionfruit plant can be dried and steeped into tea. Having a cup of tea about an hour before you're planning to sleep will help you fall asleep much faster and improve the quality of sleep you have, allowing you to wake up feeling well rested.

Chamomile

Chamomile might be even better known as a way to combat insomnia. Having a cup of chamomile tea before bedtime will calm your mind and body and help you to fall asleep much faster. While chamomile has no side effects, it is best that those who are sensitive to chrysanthemums or ragweed, rather use an alternative option to combat insomnia.

Herbal Remedies for Improved Physical Performance

Athletes and fitness enthusiasts have already been exploring ways to improve their physical performance for decades. However, more recently, this became a matter of interest to a much larger segment of the wider population. Here too, herbal remedies can be a helpful aid to increase muscle mass and strength. Plants can be a potent aid as they are loaded with several active ingredients like terpenoids, polyphenols, and alkaloids.

The herb that will contribute the most to your goals in this regard is ginseng.

Ginseng

Ginseng roots can be used as a supplement to increase endurance, but also contains active ingredients that assist with improved speed training—for example, in cycling and sprinting. Cayenne pepper, purple willow bark, and gingerroot are all options often used with ginseng.

Green Tea

Improved physical performance is only one of the many health benefits you can enjoy from having a regular cup of green tea. The active components in green tea help to ease the pain athletes experience in their joints and muscles and it will help you to get back to working out much faster after an injury.

Hormonal Health for Women

Throughout a woman's life, she goes through several severe hormonal changes. The first takes place during puberty; then, later on, it is pregnancies that place a toll on her system; and finally, it's going into menopause. Every time such a change occurs, her hormonal balance is under pressure, causing a range of concerns like being emotional, having hot flushes, breast tenderness, and more. These changes can also impact her fertility and overall health, as they are major contributing factors to oxidative stress. But Mother Nature offers her assistance in this regard too.

Ashwagandha

The herb is also known as Indian ginseng, and it belongs to the nightshade family. The plant is often used in fusions and teas and can even be used in root powder form. The herb contributes to overall well-being as it manages stress levels and because of the impact it has on the body. Women using this herb state that they enjoy better sleep and are less stressed as their blood cortisol levels drop (Snyder, 2021). *Cortisol* is the stress hormone that helps your body prepare during moments of threat but elongated exposure will cause various other health concerns.

More recent studies also indicate that the herb can impact other hormones too, like insulin and reproductive hormones (Snyder, 2021).

Marjoram

The herb is quite a common name in the kitchen and can be used in various types of food to add flavor to your favorite meals. The active components in marjoram can contribute to female wellness. It appears that a marjoram extract can lower estradiol levels in the body. This is the hormone produced by the ovaries and is linked to PCOS. As little as one cup twice a day can bring about a major improvement in this regard (Snyder, 2021).

Chaste Berry

Chaste berries are the berries of the chaste tree, also familiar to many as a "monk's pepper" or "vitex." The berries are loaded with an active component that improves dopamine levels, and they minimize the presence of prolactin in the blood. The latter is a hormone that is directly linked to premenstrual syndrome (PMS) symptoms like breast tenderness and pain.

There are also study results linking the herb to overcoming fertility challenges, and the impact of menopause (Snyder, 2021).

Hormonal Health for Men

While testosterone is a hormone present in men and women, it is especially in men's health that it plays a major role. It is responsible for sustaining several aspects of their overall health and wellness, and when testosterone levels drop, men experience a range of health concerns. Some of these concerns are fatigue, poor erectile functioning, lack of sleep, loss of body hair, and even depression.

These are all concerns that can be addressed naturally.

Ashwagandha

The herb can make a major contribution to male health too. It increases the production of testosterone, which will improve sperm health, sex drive, and sperm motility.

Pine Bark Extract

Pine bark extract improves circulation, which is often also a cause of erectile dysfunction. Furthermore, it will also improve testosterone production, which contributes to overall male wellness.

Mental Clarity and Focus

A lack of sleep, insufficient nutrient intake, poor self-care, and being overly stressed are all factors that can impact your ability to focus and maintain your concentration. In such a state, you may feel fatigued and foggy and will struggle to remember things. While it is always important to address the causes of your concern first, several herbs will improve your situation. Two very popular natural options are ginseng and guarana, but they aren't the only solutions that will bring the relief you seek.

Sage

Sage is another common name in the kitchen but it can also deliver far more benefits than merely adding flavor to food. Sage contains high levels of various active compounds that will improve alertness, memory, and mood. It is also rich in compounds that contribute to brain functioning and motivation.

Peppermint

Often enjoyed as a tea to get rid of gas buildup, peppermint is one of the most widely found herbs in homes across the globe. The plant is known for its strong aroma, an aroma that increases alertness, energy levels, and mood. Peppermint is also used to improve athletic performance and boost energy levels.

Herbs to Help You Detox

Processed foods are easy to access and a popular choice to have for a large part of the global population. As this food type needs to have a longer shelf life, these products are loaded with artificial components in the form of preservatives, colorant, and flavorings. Once consumed, these are all toxins gathering inside the body. Yet, processed foods aren't the only cause of high toxin levels in the body. Air pollution and the environment also play a major contributing role.

As it appears almost impossible to escape exposure to these toxins, it is vital to rid yourself of them regularly by detoxing. There are several ways how you can approach detoxing, and the following herbs will support your efforts.

Dandelion

Dandelion is loaded with vitamins and minerals that contribute to overall health and wellness. It is also a wonderful diuretic supporting the functioning of the liver and gallbladder. Have a cup of tea made of the roots of the plant, add the leaves to your salads, or have the flowers sautéed.

Milk Thistle

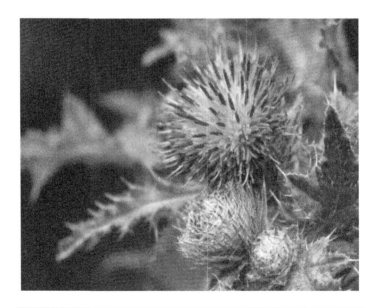

Milk thistle and liver functioning are undeniably linked and have been for ages. The plant contains *silymarin*, an active component that plays a vital role in detoxification. It helps to improve the stability of cell membranes and has an anti-inflammatory effect. Keep in mind that the active ingredient is not water-soluble and the body usually only has a very low absorption rate, so you'll have to take a stronger preparation to enjoy all the benefits it has to offer.

There are many more herbs that you can use to support overall health and wellness. But, simply by getting familiar with these herbs and building your own reference of the impact they have on you, you are creating a strong foundation to become even better acquainted with all that nature has to offer in terms of supporting holistic wellness.

Turmeric

Turmeric roots are closely related to ginger and have been at the center of Chinese and Ayurvedic medicine for centuries. The active ingredient in turmeric is *curcumin*, which is rich in anti-inflammatory and antioxidative properties, helping the body to cleanse and heal itself. Turmeric root powder is widely available, but you can also opt to use the far more potent fresh roots. When using turmeric and black pepper together, you'll add the strength of the turmeric and enjoy even more benefits from the plant.

Chapter 7:

Herbal Remedies for Cosmetic and

Hygienic Use

The contents of your apothecary are not only intended for internal healing and well-being, as it has as many uses in the world of cosmetics and in sustaining hygiene. For the longest time, the cosmetic industry has been receiving scrutiny, and, yet, it is still an industry that leaves us with a lot of questions. The greatest concern is the lack of transparency; even though labels may make statements regarding production and research, these are hardly ever worth a read.

How do cosmetic companies manage to deceive such a large part of the population? There are two reasons for this taking place. The one is that people are rather vain in general, and if we are told that using a certain product will bring greater beauty or lasting youth, the trend is to turn a blind eye to the truth behind the practices and ingredients that deliver these results. The second reason is that these companies have fat budgets that can pay for legal and marketing services that can paint a pretty picture and even make consumers believe that what they are purchasing is both good for them and safe for the environment.

Typical examples of how they do this is through wordplay. These companies are free to use words like "natural" or "organic." The FDA has never really limited the use of the word "natural." Due to the improper definition of the term, cosmetic companies can use the word according to free will, deliberately creating the impression that the product contains only natural ingredients, while it doesn't. When it comes to using the word "organic," the FDA is strict on its use when it comes to food products but is rather vague about the term when it comes to the cosmetic industry.

"Free of synthetics" is another phrase used to sell products. So, these brands are aware of the fact that many consumers of their products have made a mental link and often see synthetics in a negative light. Yet, not all synthetic products are bad and not *only* synthetic products are bad. There are many other nonsynthetics that they still add to their products which aren't good for you either, especially with long-term use.

Lastly, the following statement is as empty as the others already listed—"nontoxic," "gentle," or "hypoallergenic." There is no limitation on the use of these words and while they serve as an indication that these items are safe to use, using these words doesn't imply that the company can be held responsible in any legal matter if proven otherwise.

Even though largely ignored, these are all alarming features of the many sought-after and pricey products you'll find in the cosmetic industry.

What's the alternative? Let's see how many truly natural, gentle, and affordable solutions you can find in your apothecary.

Shampoo

To make herbal shampoo, you can take the long road or a much easier solution. The long road would be to make your own castile soap foundation and the easier solution is to just buy a quality liquid castile soap to use as the foundation for your shampoo. To this you can add any of a selection of herbal teas and blends to create the shampoo you desire, obtaining a specific outcome from each option:

- **Chamomile** is a trusted ingredient to add to shampoo when you are struggling with dandruff. The tea will leave your hair shiny and you can also expect faster hair growth.

- **Rosemary** increases circulation to the roots of your hair and as improved circulation also means that more nutrients can be absorbed, it boosts hair growth. Rosemary also takes care of hair root follicles and keeps them healthy.

- **Calendula** has many nourishing properties for the skin and does wonders for your scalp. It contains many nourishing elements that will keep your hair in a healthy condition.

Add about three tablespoons of each of these dried herbs and let the mixture steep in 1 cup of boiling water until it has reached room temperature. Combine this with ½ cup of liquid castile soap and stir well. For added benefits, you can also add ½ teaspoon of jojoba or argan oil and about 20 drops of essential oils, if you prefer.

Body Wash

Except for being soft and gentle while still enjoying all the cleansing power of nature, the other benefit of making your own herbal body wash is that it offers you the freedom to create a product that is perfectly suited to your unique needs. That said, there are certain basic ingredients that you will need to include to create a quality solution.

Once again, you'll use liquid castile soap as your foundation. To this, you can add a selection of the following natural ingredients:

- **Glycerin** is a *humectant*, meaning that it serves as a bond between the water and your skin. It also helps to moisturize the skin and is a trusted aid to improve dry skin.

- **Essential oils** fight off inflammation and keep your skin healthy. It also clears the skin of free radicals it may contain, something which contributes to aging. Another benefit of essential oils is that it even contains certain cancer-preventing properties.

- **Olive oil** adds moisture and can fight off inflammation. Only add olive oil to your body wash if you aren't already using it as part of your moisturizing routine.

- **Shea butter** is widely used in many cosmetic products due to the many benefits it contains to protect your skin from allergies, rashes, and sunburn. It is moisturizing and helps with healing. Due to all these benefits, it also plays a role in slowing down aging.

- **Almond oil** moisturizes and feeds your skin, but it also has another beneficial and rather unique trait. It loosens dead skin cells, making it easier to remove these cells and speeding up cell renewal, giving you a radiant appeal.

- **Honey** has antibacterial, anti-inflammatory, and moisturizing effects. It heals wounds and stops itching. As it helps the skin to retain its moisture, it supports a youthful appearance.

- **Coconut milk** is antibacterial and contains high levels of vitamin E, which slows down aging, and vitamin A which improves the elasticity of the skin, something we lose as we age.

Making body wash is easy. Liquid castile soap is the foundation of most natural body wash recipes and you'll need about half a cup of it. Add 2 tablespoons of glycerin and coconut oil, and 1 tablespoon of olive oil and vitamin E oil, or shea butter. Add about 20 drops of essential oil of your choice. Great options are grapefruit, lemon, or orange oil to achieve a fresh and revitalizing product. You can add all of this in a soap dispenser, shake it well, and your body wash is complete. Just remember to give it a good shake every time before use.

Moisturizer

Many plants are loaded with the most magnificent active ingredients to boost skin health, prevent aging and improve appearance. These potent components can be found in their roots, bark, petals, or leaves. You can also use fresh plant parts—for example, by harvesting aloe gel in a few easy steps from these leaves. However, dried plant parts can work as effectively, like when steeping chamomile flowers to add to your beauty products.

Making an herbal moisturizer at home is easy and would only require a few ingredients. What you'll get in return though is an effective product that will care for your skin without any added chemicals.

Argan, lavender, jasmine, and rose oil do wonders for dry skin, while sandalwood and geranium oils are good choices for normal skin. People with oily skin will enjoy the benefits of grape-seed oil, jojoba, tea tree, or any citrus-based oil.

Use two tablespoons of aloe vera gel and add five to six drops of any vegetable or nut oil to it. I'll suggest that you try almond oil, but experiment with other oils too to see which works the best for you. Mix it up well before adding five drops of essential oil of your choice and one to two drops of lavender oil—or any other oil—to add fragrance. Add two to three drops of vitamin E oil; if you prefer to add glycerin, you can also add one to two drops to the mixture. Mix it all well until smooth paste forms and your moisturizer is complete. It is best to keep this in a cool, dark place and use it within a month.

Wrinkles

Whether wrinkles are something you wear with grace or consider to be your worst nightmare, most of us try to slow down aging for as long as we can. Luckily, there are many ways to address wrinkles by using only natural ingredients.

Olive oil is a great base to massage into your skin at the affected areas as it helps to tighten the skin. You can add using a face mask to this routine. Mash an avocado and let this sit on your skin for about 20 minutes to tighten the skin while it also replenishes the oil. Another option is to mix about 1 tablespoon of lemon juice with a few drops of vitamin E oil and natural yogurt. You can allow this mask to sit for about 20 minutes before washing it off. While these are all ways to address wrinkles externally, drinking ginger tea regularly will combat wrinkles from the inside.

Makeup Remover

Olive and coconut oil are both effective ways to remove even the most stubborn makeup from your skin while serving as a moisturizing agent too. If you prefer to use something less oily, you can also use cucumber juice or even milk.

Chapped lips

Chapped lips can be painful and don't compliment your appearance. It is a concern most of us face during the cold of winter, but it can also be the result of exposure to any other natural elements like the sun or wind. Other causes of chapped lips are vitamin deficiency, dehydration, or even exposure to irritants like toothpaste. While you can apply coconut oil, you may want to add something to the oil to speed up healing. So, use coconut oil as a carrier oil—to which you can add grape-seed or tea tree oil—to see a faster improvement.

Dry Skin

There are so many things that can cause your skin to become excessively dry, even to the point where it starts to get inflamed and be very sensitive. Olive oil and coconut oil will both bring relief to dry skin, but you can also choose to use either as a carrier oil to which you can add even more great natural ingredients. Vitamin E oil does wonders for dry skin, and you only need to add a few drops to a carrier oil to improve your condition.

To clear dry skin and boost cell renewal by getting rid of dead skin cells, you can make a scrub of sugar and coconut oil. For added richness, you can apply an avocado mask afterward.

Stretch Marks

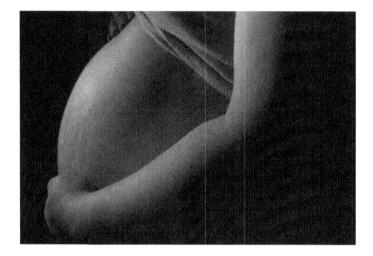

Stretch marks are usually synonymous with pregnancy, but there are also other contributing factors to this skin condition that may leave you feeling self-conscious. Rather than trying expensive products burdened with chemicals, apply coconut oil to the affected area. Coconut oil contains fatty acids that are easily absorbed by the skin and it will speed up recovery. You can also try aloe vera gel or cocoa butter. While lemon juice may not repair the skin, it will lighten the appearance of the affected area and improve the way it looks.

Dark Eye Circles

You may be familiar with the benefit of leaving cucumber slices on your eyes to get rid of the dark circles, but this isn't the only natural way to shed these circles. Crush a couple of mint leaves and apply this onto the affected area to get rid of these circles to leave your skin looking radiant and fresh. Another natural solution is to leave aloe vera pulp on these dark spots for about 10 minutes before washing it off.

Body Odor

Body odor can be caused by a range of concerns. Natural ways to combat bad breath are to brush your teeth with baking soda. This will neutralize the smell and can fight off bacteria causing the odor. You can also chew on caraway, anise, dill, or fennel to improve your breath.

The risk of using deodorants is widely underpublished. You would apply these products that are full of chemicals to the most sensitive skin areas, and, yet, the risk of all the toxins your body absorbs may be completely unknown to you. However, bad body odor isn't the only alternative. Mix ½ cup of apple cider vinegar with ½ cup of water into a spritz. Apply this to your underarms. The smell of the vinegar disappears within minutes, but its bacteria-fighting properties remain active for hours, preventing bacteria from causing any nasty odors. You can also make your own roll-on at home. Combine ¼ cup of baking soda, ½ cup of cornstarch, and a few drops of your preferred essential oils before adding 3 tablespoons of coconut oil. You can then mix it into a paste. Fill up an empty roll-on dispenser and apply as per usual.

Fight stinky feet by adding ½ cup of baking soda or table salt to a bucket of hot water and soak your feet for half an hour. If the smell is caused by athletes' feet you can add 20–30 drops of tea tree oil to your bath to enjoy relief from this concern.

Cellulite

While increasing your water intake will help to flush out the toxins causing cellulite, you can improve results by making a coffee scrub to apply to the affected area. Mix a ¼ cup of coffee grounds, 3 tablespoons of brown sugar, and 3 tablespoons of coconut oil together. Use this to scrub the area for a couple of minutes before washing it off. Repeat this 3 times a week to enjoy optimal results.

You can also massage the area with a mixture of one part apple cider vinegar and two parts water to which you've added a few drops of honey.

Dandruff

Tea tree oil in your shampoo will combat dandruff, but if you have specific problematic spots on your scalp, you can add tea tree oil directly to these areas. Aloe gel will also work. Just apply the gel directly as squeezed from the leaves.

Hair growth

Again, you can add oils to your shampoo that will encourage growth, or you can add a few drops of oil to a carrier oil and massage this into your scalp. Good carrier oils to use for this purpose are coconut, jojoba, olive, wheat germ, or sweet almond oil. To these, you can add Brahmi, ginseng, or Chinese hibiscus to encourage hair growth.

Scarring

Whether it is from acne or injury, scarring—especially when it is on your face—can affect your self-confidence. The following natural ingredients can improve the appearance of scars. Apply aloe vera gel to the scarred area and massage it into your skin. Let it sit on the scar for 30 minutes before rinsing it off. Repeat this twice daily.

You can also massage vitamin E oil into the area for 10 minutes and then leave it on for another 20 minutes before washing it off. Do this 3 times daily. Rubbing lemon juice in the area will improve its appearance. Rug it in for a couple of minutes and then let it sit for 10 minutes before washing it off. Try to repeat this daily at the same time.

Toothpaste

What are the ingredients you need to make natural toothpaste at home?

Clay to cleanse the teeth and sea salt for its antibacterial and whitening properties. Sage, cinnamon, cloves, and peppermint can all add flavor and increase healing inside the mouth. Neem will help to clean the teeth and stevia will improve the taste.

For the base of your natural toothpaste, mix together baking soda, bentonite clay, and finely ground calcium powder. To this, you can add sea salt, ground sage, spirulina, neem, or essential oils like peppermint. Lastly, add water, coconut oil, or liquid castile soap. This recipe leaves you with a lot of freedom to add what you prefer and to mix as much as you desire into a paste that has the consistency you like.

All-Purpose Cleaner

The best all-purpose cleaner that will get rid of any kind of dirt without damaging your surfaces or naturally consists of only three ingredients. Add ½ cup of white vinegar, 2 tablespoons of baking soda, and 10 drops of essential oil of your choice into a spray bottle. Shake it up and use it as necessary.

The number of natural alternatives to beauty and hygiene is offering you a vast range to choose from. Yet, the best feature is still not the fact that these ingredients are widely available or much more affordable than commercially sold solutions, but that it contains only natural goodness without exposing yourself to chemicals and toxins.

Chapter 8:

How to Make Your Own Essential Oils

From Scratch

When you are just starting out with your apothecary, you may want to purchase essential oils rather than making your own, and there is nothing wrong with that as long as you invest your money in buying only oils of high quality. However, you'll soon discover that essential oils can be rather pricey, and they can become a steep investment if you want to expand the collection of oils in your stock. Therefore, making your essential oils at home is the solution many herbalists prefer. In this chapter, I am sharing exactly how you can do this, but I also want to explain the difference between essential oils and infused oils.

Essential Oils Compared to Infused Oils

The most prominent difference between the two oils is that infused oils are much easier to make than essential oils. While the latter requires distillation, *infused oils* are merely the result of the process of soaking the herbs of your choice in a carrier oil. For example, you can soak lavender, or calendula, in oil and you'll have a wonderful end product containing many properties that support healing. However, it is not as potent as essential oils, and, therefore, you may want to try your hand at making your own essential oils.

Oil Extraction

Oil extraction refers to the process of extracting oil from plants that don't naturally come across as oily. Peppermint oil is one such example. Peppermint leaves don't appear to be oily, and yet they contain oil that you can extract. Just take note that you'll need a lot of leaves to extract a sufficient amount of oil.

For this, you'll need a Crock-Pot and lid; distilled water; and a lot of plant material like leaves or flowers. Decide what plant you are going to use to extract oil from. You are also free to use a combination of plants to create a blend. Add the plant material to the pot and cover it with water. Make sure that you don't exceed three quarters of the pot's capacity. Put the lid on upside down. Turn the heat on high until the water is hot. Then, reduce the heat and allow the pot to simmer for three to four hours until all the plant material is cooked down. Allow the contents to cool down before putting it all inside the fridge. Once a thin layer of oil forms on the surface, you need to scoop this off as this is the oil you've extracted. You'll have to be quick because it quickly melts, and then you'll have to refrigerate the pot again. This layer of oil is what you want to keep as it is the oil extracted from the plant. As one final step to get rid of any water that might have gotten into the oil you've scooped off is to heat up the oil again to allow the water to evaporate. But, be careful as the longer the oil is exposed to heat, the more of its potent properties it will lose. Keep the oil in a cool dark place in an airtight bottle.

Tips for Oil Extraction

The following tips will help you to enjoy the best results when extracting essential oils:

- You can use dried herbs, but fresh herbs are better as they contain more oils.

- The best time to harvest these herbs is early in the morning just after their leaves dried off any dew. Different plants also have different stages when they contain higher volumes of oil. Do proper research to determine when the best stage is to harvest the plants from which you want to extract oil.

- Harvest at least four cups of plant material to get a couple of teaspoons of oil.

- Increase the plant surface exposed to allow for a better extraction ratio by chopping up your herbs.

- Always use distilled water. Tap water contains bacteria and chemicals which you don't want in contact with your oil.

Benefits of Essential Oils

As essential oils are so potent, you'll only need a few drops—often added to a quality carrier oil—to enjoy a range of benefits. The benefits you access by using these oils range from hormone management to improved cognitive functioning.

Hormone Management

The essential oils from thyme, sage, and geranium are known for their ability to bring progesterone and estrogen levels in balance. Therefore, they are used to improve PCOS and the symptoms linked to PMS and menopause.

Other essential oils help to reduce cortisol levels. It is how it can support stress management and even improves the symptoms of depression.

Better Digestion

Ginger oil relieves constipation, indigestion, and the symptoms of ulcers. Some oils help to stimulate the release of digestive enzymes which improves digestion and nutrient uptake. Essential oils are also trusted to improve diarrhea, stomach spasms, and irritable bowel syndrome (IBS).

Pain Relief

You'll find pain relief by using the oils of pepper, marjoram, peppermint, and lavender. Other oils that are working wonders to bring you the relief you seek are chamomile, thyme, marjoram, rosemary, frankincense, and eucalyptus.

Address Headaches and Migraines

As essential oils improve circulation and reduce stress, they are addressing the cause of many headaches and migraines rather than just bringing relief to the symptoms. It is especially lavender oil that is linked as an aid in this regard, as you only have to sniff the aroma of the oil for a couple of minutes to experience pain relief (Axe, 2021).

Better Sleep

Smelling the scent of lavender is so relaxing and soothing that it will help you to sleep. Other helpful oils are chamomile, bergamot, and ylang-ylang.

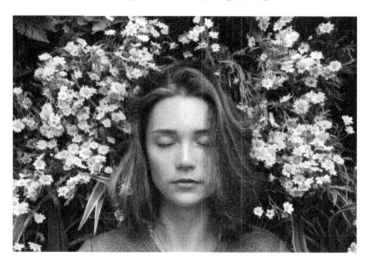

Detox Support

As oils help to improve digestion, you can also use them to rid your body of toxins. Fennel, lemon, lemongrass, ginger, and grapefruit oil are all helpful in this regard.

A Mood Booster

Due to the strong aroma of these oils, they play in on our olfactory senses which can improve your overall mood. Essential oils that are especially helpful in reducing anxiety are bergamot, frankincense, rose, ylang-ylang, and orange.

Skin and Hair Support

Throughout this book, we've discussed several herbs that support hair and skin health. You can apply the oils of a more potent solution to address your concerns. Oils that are linked to hair and skin health are lavender, tea tree, frankincense, myrrh, sage, and rosemary.

Strengthen Your Immunity

Many essential oils contain potent antiviral, antiseptic, antifungal, and anti-inflammatory properties, and, therefore, these oils can be used to fight infection. Try oregano, eucalyptus, ginger, lemon, cinnamon, or frankincense to boost your immune system.

Better Cognitive Functioning

Essential oils fight off free radicals that contribute to the deterioration experienced by those who suffer from cognitive function disorders like Alzheimer's disease. These oils can also be used to improve learning, focus, and memory. Those who suffer from dementia also often suffer from higher levels of agitation and you can also use essential oils to ease these symptoms. The essential oils mostly linked to these outcomes are jasmine, lavender, and eucalyptus.

Boosting Your Energy Levels

Like with your mood, smelling certain essential oils will also boost your energy levels and improve your focus. The options that are most trusted in this regard are lemongrass, grapefruit, eucalyptus, and lemon. Another way to reap this benefit is by adding a couple of drops of peppermint oil to a glass of water. The oil increases brain oxygen which improves concentration.

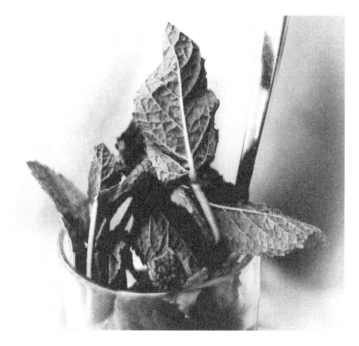

The Top 15 Essential Oils

There are so many essential oils to choose from that it can be confusing to know where you need to start when you first begin building your apothecary. While it will be beneficial to research what oils will address your unique concerns best and then stock up on these oils, the following oils are widely considered to be the most popular choices to have in your collection:

- **Peppermint** improves headaches, pain, fever, digestion, and energy levels.

- **Eucalyptus** does wonders to open airways and for easy breathing when suffering from allergies, colds, sinusitis, or bronchitis.

- **Ginger** improves digestion and relieves nausea, but it also soothes pain and inflammation in muscles and joints.

- **Lavender** helps to soothe your mood and brings a sense of calm supporting sleep. It can also treat cuts and wounds or even burns.

- **Clove oil** is antibacterial and antiparasitic, and it offers antioxidant protection.

- **Frankincense** supports the immune system, improves age spots, can fight off inflammation, and even combat some types of cancer.

- **Rosemary oil** improves hair thickness and brain function, making it a popular choice for shampoos and to improve your ability to study or work alike.

- **Cypress** reduces varicose veins as it supports healthy circulation. It also plays a role in healing bone fractures much faster.

- **Grapefruit** can give your metabolism the boost it needs, and it can clear up cellulite.

- **Rose oil** added to your moisturizer will leave you with a radiant appeal as it eases inflammation in the skin. Rose oil can reduce skin inflammation, and it's great for creating glowing skin. Enrich your moisturizer with a couple of drops.

- **Lemon oil** is an essential ingredient of effective homemade cleaning products due to its antibacterial properties.

- **Myrrh** is another natural antiseptic, and, while not so commonly used in cleaning products, it can prevent infection and inflammation of the skin.

- **Oregano oil** is antimicrobial, antifungal, and antimicrobial, making it a trusted partner when combatting most diseases.

- **Tea tree oil** can also do wonders in fighting off disease, supporting the immune system, and even preventing odors due to its high natural antibacterial and antifungal.

- **Sandalwood** is a natural aphrodisiac and is often used as a remedy to improve libido.

If you stock up on these essential oils, you will be able to treat a wide range of concerns. However, these are only the oils that will provide you with a strong foundation to expand your collection with many more oils that are applicable to your unique situation and the concerns you aim to address through the use of essential oils.

Chapter 9:

How to Make Raw Herbal Teas

Herbal teas are healing in a cup. Yes, just by drinking a comforting cup of tea made with a potent blend of dried herbs, you will be able to enjoy a wide range of health benefits. When you are making tea blends, you'll be using different parts of the herbs in your garden. For some plants, you'll be steeping the leaves like the mint family, while for others, you'll be using roots, seeds, or flowers.

If you've dried your herbs following the correct methods as discussed earlier on and have stuck to the storage guidelines to improve the longevity of these dried herbs, you'll be able to blend your teas easily and can even store already made-up blends ready for use. As always, be sure to label your blends correctly, including listing the ingredients in the jar, as well as the necessary dates.

Steeping Tea

Many people are unsure about what is the correct method to steep tea, but this is mostly due to the rushed lifestyle most live. Thus, we only steep prepared tea bags strung onto a tag, leaving the art of steeping loose-leaf tea largely forgotten. So, let's step back in time and get familiar with the proper way of steeping herbal tea.

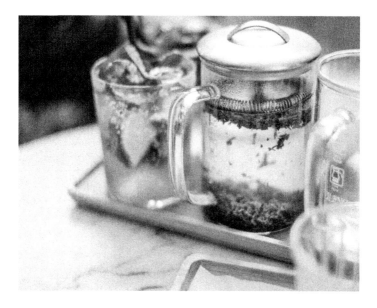

To steep tea, you would need to put your leaves, boiling water, a tea strainer, and a teapot. Add the boiling water to the leaves and let them sit for about 15 minutes. Only then is your tea going to be strong enough as it's given sufficient time for the potent ingredients in the herbs to infuse with the water. Typically, you'll use about ½ teaspoon of dried herbs per cup of tea you are making. While most herbal tea blends are made of dried herbs, you can also use fresh herbs. The process is much the same, but you'll need about 3 times as many herbs as when using them dry. While the tea blend would predominantly consist of herbs, you can also add additional flavorings to make the tea tastier. Herbalists would often use dried fruit bits or honey to bring additional flavor to their cups.

Tea Recipes to Keep in Your Apothecary

As the herbalist in charge of your apothecary, you have the freedom to experiment with different blends. But, when you are new to alternative healing, you may feel unsure about where to start. The following herbal tea recipes will help to guide you and help you find your feet when it comes to blending teas that are tasty and potent in their healing capabilities.

Flu-Fighting Blend

In this blend, you'll combine the fighting power of lemon and elderflowers to create a tasty tea that will ease the symptoms of colds and flu.

Use one teaspoon of elderflowers. For this blend, you can use dried flowers, but if you have fresh flowers available, you can use them too. Add no more than two teaspoons of lemon juice and one teaspoon of honey. Add boiling water and let it steep until room temperature.

Relaxing and Soothing Tea Blend

By now, you are aware of the soothing qualities present in the active compound found in lavender. Add to that the antibacterial properties of mint, and you have a blend that is calming and improves your digestion while fighting off infection.

Use 1 teaspoon of dried mint leaves and ¼ teaspoon of lavender flowers. Add 1 teaspoon of honey to add a bit of healthy sweetness, and fill the cup with boiling water. You can have this tea hot or cold.

Tasty Apple Cinnamon Tea

The beauty of using natural ingredients is often in the fact that you need so few ingredients to create a solution that is tasty and effective. For this tea, you'll only need 1 tablespoon of dried apple pieces and ½ tablespoon of crushed cinnamon sticks. For an even healthier choice, you can use organic apples. Add boiling water and let it sit. This tea also works equally well as a warm, soothing drink or as a refreshing, chilled drink.

Benefits of Herbal Teas

You know that herbal teas have healing properties, but what specific concerns can you treat in this manner? The following are only some treatment solutions you'll be able to enjoy from herbal tea blends.

Relief of Stress and Anxiety

A blend of kava root, Saint-John's-wort, chamomile, valerian, and chamomile will boost your mood and energy, improve the symptoms of depression and reduce the risk of inflammation. It also contributes to preventing chronic diseases.

Combat Insomnia

Several herbs have sedative properties. A perfect blend to have before heading off to bed includes kava root, lavender, valerian, and chamomile.

Keep Chronic Disease at Bay

There is a wide range of chronic diseases that can place a toll on your overall health and wellness, while also draining you mentally and emotionally. At best, you want to keep them at bay and the herbal tea blend that will help you with this includes dandelion, peppermint, cinnamon, chamomile, and, of course, ginger.

Boost Immune Defense

Elderberry, licorice, lemon, ginger, and echinacea are all herbs that contain high levels of antioxidants to help your body defend itself against disease. Therefore, regularly indulge yourself with a cup of these blends during cold and flu seasons.

Analgesic Relief

Tea blends that will help you to overcome discomfort and recover from surgery, injury, or even illness include herbs like chamomile, bergamot, kava root, allspice, and eucalyptus.

Better Digestion

Poor digestion doesn't only impact the body's ability to enjoy proper nutrient uptake, but it can also cause discomfort and pain. Drinking a blend that contains cinnamon, ginger, peppermint, dandelion, and chamomile can ease nausea and vomiting; stomach cramps; bloating; diarrhea; indigestion; and cramps.

Brain Boosting Blends

There are times when we can all do with a bit better focus and lasting concentration. If you are struggling with either, have a cup of mint, rooibos, dandelion, ginger, or rose hip tea.

Stop Inflammation From Spreading

Whether you are experiencing inflammation in your joints or muscles—or even in the form of stomach cramps—it is painful or discomforting, at the very least. You'll find some relief from these symptoms by drinking a cup of turmeric, eucalyptus, ginger, or peppermint tea.

Detox

Several herbs contain potent diuretic or laxative properties. These herbs will help your body to clear itself of toxins and to enjoy healthier living. When you detox, it is the liver, kidneys, and gastrointestinal system that are under severe pressure. Hibiscus, juniper, green, and hawthorn tea blends can all bring some welcome relief in this regard.

The Top 15 Teas to Stock Up

What are the teas that are the most beneficial to have in your apothecary? The most accurate answer to this will be teas that are directed at treating the medical concerns you and your family are battling with the most. However, this is not only true when it comes to teas but also to tinctures, essential oils, or oil infusions. That said, the following 15 teas address the most common health concerns and, therefore, are the popular choices to be included in any apothecary:

- **Peppermint** tea improves a wide range of digestive concerns from indigestion to stomach aches and getting rid of excess gas that can often be painful to endure. Furthermore, it also contributes to immune support.

- **Chamomile** tea helps to calm the nerves and is a soothing drink to have before bedtime. It also improves pain often caused by inflammation or arthritis. Its healing properties help improve skin concerns like sunburn or any other form of skin irritation.

- **Rooibos** tea has many healing properties from calming your mood to improving headaches, high blood pressure, allergic responses, and skin disorders. It is a tea linked with lasting youth.

- **Ginger** is a wonderful aid to combat nausea and digestion will improve appetite. It also fights certain chronic diseases.

- **Anise** tea, like ginger, addresses several digestive concerns but it also brings relief to menstrual cramps and can fight off colds.

- **Dandelion** is a diuretic that clears the body of toxins due to increased urination. It also lowers blood pressure and can be used to address iron deficiency.

- **Thyme** tea boosts the immune system, fights fever, and improves cold symptoms like coughing. It can also bring pain relief to headaches.

- **Turmeric** tea contains curcumin which brings about several healing properties like it fighting inflammation and even certain types of cancer. It is also a wonderful antioxidant and improves digestion.

- **Echinacea** tea is a superhero when it comes to fighting infection. It boosts the immune system and also gets rid of inflammation, both inside the body and on the surface.

- **Cannabis** tea eases anxiety, depression, stress, and headaches, as well as inflammation, pain, and indigestion.

- **Patchouli** tea strengthens the immune system and detoxes the body, but it also improves mood and increases libido.

- **Valerian** root tea eases spasms and lowers stress levels, and it also has sedative properties that will help you to enjoy quality sleep.

- **Kava root** tea, much like valerian root tea, helps to ease stress and anxiety and, therefore, supports quality sleep. Furthermore, you can also use it to detox the body.

- **Rose hip** tea contains high levels of vitamin C and is, therefore, great at fighting off infection and supporting the immune system. This tea will also detox the body.

- **Osmanthus** tea treats coughs, and congestion; it clears the body of toxins; and helps to get rid of bad breath.

Possible Side Effects

It is quite ironic how easily the wider population will swallow anything that is a prescription, often without pondering on the side effects they are exposing themselves to. Yet, they may be very wary of side effects when offered herbal alternatives.

While most herbal solutions don't have any side effects, you may have to be aware of the following side effects linked to herbal teas. These effects are only present due to the high level of potent ingredients present in herbs.

Allergies

Herbs are plants, so some people may show allergic reactions to some of the herbs we've discussed. If you are allergic to a specific plant, you'll likely experience symptoms like diarrhea, skin rashes, nausea, vomiting, stomach cramps, and finding it hard to breathe. If you are concerned that you may be allergic to a specific herb, it is best to discuss your concerns with a qualified herbalist.

Toxic When Consumed in Large Quantities

Some herbs have healing properties, but, if you overdo them, the active components may have an adverse effect. Some herbs can be toxic if consumed in large quantities. Examples of such herbs are comfrey and foxglove. It can also be that you've misidentified a specific herb while harvesting, as some herbs do look very similar to toxic plants. Therefore, it is best to always be sure that you've correctly identified the herbs you are taking home. This is even more so the case when you are planning on using these herbs for teas or tisanes.

Interaction With Prescription

While some herbs may be completely harmless, the active ingredients they have to offer may interact with the medication you are already taking. Therefore, it is best to get professional advice first if you are planning on combining herbal and conventional treatment options.

Overuse

If a little of something is good, then more of it must be better, right? No, when you are advised to drink only half a cup of tea from a specific blend, then sticking to that and taking no more for moderation are often key to your success. Some teas can be so potent that if you consume too much, it can have an adverse impact on your overall well-being.

While these side effects are surely a matter that should be taken seriously, it is also important to know that it is mostly the case that people don't experience any side effects from using herbal blends. What these side effects also confirm is that herbal teas are a potent alternative to conventional medicine and that these teas truly hold the power to establish healing.

Conclusion

Many centuries ago, humankind had only one solution to treat ailments and support overall wellness. Then, the world became more civilized, and, to a large degree, we've convinced ourselves that we are also growing more intelligent. This belief is true to a certain degree as, sure, we have access to solutions today that our ancestors didn't even dream about. But what does true intelligence really mean? While we are surely making progress in certain regards, our ability to be independent and rely on natural resources to sustain ourselves have been crippled.

At the center of this process of deterioration, we find nothing but an interconnected web of lies and make-beliefs pushed by a minority for whom the health and wellness of the majority is merely an opportunity to gain profit—Big Pharma. This is why the pharmaceutical industry has reached a magnitude of wealth worth billions of dollars. It is also why we expose ourselves, our loved ones, and our children to pharmaceuticals that are riddled with chemicals. Sure, these prescription solutions can bring about healing, but at what price?

The price of severe side effects? This is a concern often brushed underneath the carpet, as it claims the lives of thousands every year; this is only in the United States, an issue that is much larger on a global scale.

The price of unaffordability? The high cost of medical care is a global concern, making health care too expensive for individuals or even communities. Even in our modern age, we still have entire villages where health care is entirely inaccessible.

Does hearing these facts leave you feeling powerless, trapped, and even angry?

This book has a dual purpose. The first is to convey the message that you don't have to buy into this culture. If the situations above describe the norm you are used to, it is also important to know that you don't have to remain stuck in the belief that only prescription drugs bring about healing. If you are one of the many people who are opting out of this system to seek alternative ways to care for the wellness of your loved ones and yourself, then this book is your guide that will direct you on this journey.

The second purpose is to share sufficient knowledge regarding herbal medicine to overcome that sense of being daunted by your lacking knowledge in this regard. After all, it is often the lack of knowledge that contributes to the sense of being trapped. So, I've taken meticulous care to share with you every aspect of herbalism, from harvesting herbs to growing your own. You now know how to dry herbs, store them, and label them correctly. You know how to make tinctures, fusions, tea blends and can extract essential oils yourself. You know what herbs to stock in your apothecary and what teas to drink to treat specific conditions but also to improve your health and wellness.

While the journey of herbalism is never completed, I've provided you with a strong foundation to spread your wings in this area with great confidence. I've provided you with a wealth of information, all compiled into one resource to make it easy to find your way. Sometimes, when you are seeking answers, it is a case that we may not even know what the questions are that we need to ask. Now you know. You know who to turn to and you know why you are ready to make this change.

You are now one of the thousands of people who said, "No more." You are now one of those who are no longer buying into a system that doesn't care about their well-being, who realizes the immense potential that nature has to offer to sustain their wellness, to treat medical concerns, and to do so effectively. You are now ready to start building your home apothecary.

If you find yourself amped to make the necessary changes and are convinced that herbal remedies should never be considered to be a second-rate approach to health and wellbeing, please promote this cause and share a positive review to get more people on board with natural healing.

Spreading the Wonderful practice of Natural Medicine

Now that you have everything you need to start your natural medicine journey, it's time to pass on your love for the practice and show other readers where they can find the same guidance.

Simply by leaving your honest opinion of this book on Amazon, you'll guide other people down the path of natural healing. Whether it be a few words or a detailed passage, leaving a review helps tremendously.

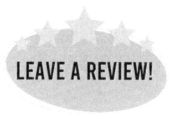

Scan one of the QR codes below to leave a review:

US   **UK**

Glossary

- **Ayurvedic medicine**: A type of alternative healing based on a holistic approach toward caring for the body, mind, and spirit that originated in India and relies on the use of herbal remedies, a healthy diet, exercise, physical therapy, and breathing techniques.

- **Carrier oils**: High-quality oils, like coconut oil, that are used for blending essential oils to dilute the potent power of the latter.

- **Curcumin**: A natural anti-inflammatory compound present in turmeric.

- **Decoction**: A very potent herbal tea infusion.

- **Diuretic**: A natural or manufactured remedy to increase urination that's often used to support detoxing the body.

- **Glycerite**: An herbal remedy relying on glycerin to extract active compounds from plant material.

- **Hardiness zone**: Refers to the specific climate in a region classified on the Hardiness Zone map based on the lowest average temperature of the area.

- **Hori hori**: A Japanese gardening tool used to dig, but it can also double up to cut roots.

- **Humectant**: A substance that helps to retain moisture.

- **190-proof grain alcohol**: A pure form of alcohol, containing about 95% alcohol by volume.

- **Paleolithic era**: Refers to a certain era in the Stone Age taking place roughly 2.5 million years ago. It was a time before the start of agriculture and humans relied on nature as their only resource.

- **Polycystic ovary syndrome (PCOS)**: A condition referring to several problems linked to the female reproductive system.

- **Poultice**: A soft mass or spread that is slightly warmed and spread onto fabric before applying as a treatment for sores or lesions.

- **Rhizome**: Plant stems that grow underneath the soil surface, from which nodes, buds, and roots can grow.

- **Silymarin**: A compound found in milk thistle with potent antioxidant properties.

- **Tincture**: Potent herbal medicine, made using alcohol to extract the active compounds from plant material.

- **Tisane**: Herbal tea made from a blend of herbs, flowers, spices, and leaves used as an alternative medicine.

References

A, J. (2019, January 18). *13 natural remedies for diaper rash (that really work!).* Expert Home Tips. https://experthometips.com/natural-remedies-for-diaper-rash

Adamant, A. (2019, September 24). *Homemade herbal shampoo recipe.* Practical Self Reliance. https://practicalselfreliance.com/herbal-shampoo/

Adelmann, M. (2013, March 27). *The herbal healing practices of Native Americans.* Herbal Academy. https://theherbalacademy.com/the-herbal-healing-practices-of-native-americans/

Alleman, G. P. (n.d.). *Herbal remedies for diarrhea.* How Stuff Works. https://health.howstuffworks.com/wellness/natural-medicine/herbal-remedies/herbal-remedies-for-diarrhea.htm

Almanza, A. (2022, April 14). *11 natural remedies for hair loss to try at home.* Reader's Digest. https://www.readersdigest.ca/health/conditions/hair-loss-natural-remedies/

Amro, M. S., Teoh, S. L., Norzana, A. G., & Srijit, D. (2018). The potential role of herbal products in the treatment of Parkinson's disease. *La Clinica Terapeutica*, *169*(1), e23–e33. https://doi.org/10.7417/T.2018.2050

Anderson, T. (2019, May 25). *Ways to use plants in herbal skincare*. Lovely Greens. https://lovelygreens.com/make-herbal-skincare-homegrown-herbs-flowers/

Anderson, L. A. (2022, August 10). *Prescription drug addiction: Top facts for you and your family*. Drugs.com. https://www.drugs.com/slideshow/prescriptio n-drug-addiction-1075

Angioedema. (n.d.). Anticoagulation Europe. https://www.anticoagulationeurope.org/conditi ons/angioedema/

ANNE. (2017, May 1). *23 medicinal plants the Native Americans used on a daily basis*. Ask a Prepper. https://www.askaprepper.com/23-medicinal-plants-native-americans-used-daily-basis/

Axe, J. (2021, October 5). *Essential oils: 11 main benefits and 101 uses*. Dr. Axe. https://draxe.com/essential-oils/essential-oil-uses-benefits/

Ayurveda. (2023, February 14). In *Wikipedia*. https://en.wikipedia.org/wiki/Ayurveda

BBC Gardeners World Magazine. (2019, January 14). *How to grow herbs.* https://www.gardenersworld.com/how-to/grow-plants/how-to-grow-herbs/

BBC Gardeners' World Magazine. (2020, April 7). *How to grow rosemary.* https://www.gardenersworld.com/how-to/grow-plants/how-to-grow-rosemary/

Belle: University Chancellor. (2022, November 2). *12 home remedies for sunburns.* Parents. https://www.parents.com/kids/safety/outdoor/sunburn-remedies/

Berry, J. (2017, November 20). *How to get rid of bruises: 7 effective home remedies.* Medical News Today. https://www.medicalnewstoday.com/articles/320090

Berry, J. (2022, December 14). *Top 16 natural remedies for eczema.* Medical News Today. https://www.medicalnewstoday.com/articles/324228

Bhatia, J. (2016, February 10). *Herbal remedies for natural pain relief.* Everyday Health. https://www.everydayhealth.com/pain-management/natural-pain-remedies.aspx

Boyles, M. (2020, June 18). *Natural ways to tame body odors.* Almanac.

https://www.almanac.com/natural-ways-tame-body-odors

Burns, C. (2018, January 11). *"Natural" or "organic" cosmetics? Don't trust marketing claims.* Environmental Working Group. https://www.ewg.org/news-insights/news/natural-or-organic-cosmetics-dont-trust-marketing-claims

Cadman, B. (2020, January 31). *10 home remedies for varicose veins.* Medical News Today. https://www.medicalnewstoday.com/articles/3 21703

Caldwell, P. (n.d.). *Storage of your herbal products.* Herb Lore. https://herblore.com/overviews/storage-of-your-herbal-products

Chatterjee, S. (2018a, September 10). S*uffering from sepsis? These home remedies will help you heal.* The Health Site. https://www.thehealthsite.com/home-remedies/601310suffering-from-sepsis-these-home-remedies-will-help-you-heal-sc0918-601310/

Chatterjee, S. (2018b, November 24). *Top 9 ways to cure measles naturally.* The Health Site. https://www.thehealthsite.com/diseases-conditions/top-9-ways-to-cure-measles-naturally-626253/

Cherney, K. (2022, October 21). *8 home remedies for acid reflux/GERD.* Healthline. https://www.healthline.com/health/gerd/home-remedies

Cherney, K. (2023, January 12). *13 natural dry-skin remedies you can DIY at home.* Everyday Health. https://www.everydayhealth.com/skin-and-beauty/natural-skin-remedies.aspx

Chilson, M. (2014, October 12). *Holistic medicine: 5 examples of cultures where it rules.* Newsmax. https://www.newsmax.com/FastFeatures/holistic-medicine-cultures/2014/10/12/id/597222/

Chinese medicine and herbs 101: A brief history. (2021, February 25). Chi-nese. https://chinese.com/chinese-medicine-and-herbs-101-a-brief-history/

Chiropractic Economics. (2013, August 21). *Naturally relieve leg cramps with herbs.* https://www.chiroeco.com/naturally-relieve-leg-cramps-with-herbs/

Cleveland Clinic. (2021, November 17). *5 best and worst home remedies for your hemorrhoids.* https://health.clevelandclinic.org/how-to-get-rid-of-hemorrhoids/

Chronic fatigue syndrome. (n.d.). St. Luke's Hospital. https://www.stlukes-stl.com/health-content/medicine/33/000035.htm

Cleversley, K. (2013, November 25). *How to make essential oils from scratch at home.* Essential Oil Exchange. https://blog.essentialoilexchange.com/how-to-make-essential-oils-from-scratch-at-home/

Codekas, C. (2016, August 5). *6 tips for storing dried herbs.* Herbal Academy. https://theherbalacademy.com/6-tips-for-storing-dried-herbs/

Cold-Q. (n.d.). *Benefits of herbal medicine you need to know.* https://coldq.com/benefits-of-herbal-medicine-you-need-to-know/

Complementary and alternative medicine pertussis. (n.d.). St. Luke's Hospital. https://www.stlukes-stl.com/health-content/medicine/33/000128.htm

Creating your home herbal apothecary. (n.d.). Mountain Rose Herbs. https://blog.mountainroseherbs.com/creating-your-home-herbal-apothecary

Crichton-Stuart, C. (2018, June 14). *What are some home remedies for shingles?* Medical News Today.

https://www.medicalnewstoday.com/articles/3
22131

Croup herbal treatment. (n.d.). McDowell's Herbal Treatments. https://www.mcdowellsherbal.com/human-conditions/childhood/92-croup-herbal-treatment

Curtis, L. (2021, May 21). *Natural remedies for lyme disease.* Verywell Health. https://www.verywellhealth.com/natural-remedies-for-lyme-disease-5180854

Cutolo, M. (2021, May 14). *13 natural gout remedies for pain and swelling you can try.* Reader's Digest, The Healthy. https://www.thehealthy.com/arthritis/gout-natural-remedies/

de Give, T. (2018, July 6). *Make your own herbal tea blends.* EatingWell. https://www.eatingwell.com/article/290911/make-your-own-herbal-tea-blends/

DoctorNDTV. (2018, May 10). *Living with lupus: 8 best home remedies for lupus.* New Delhi Television. https://www.ndtv.com/health/living-with-lupus-8-best-home-remedies-for-lupus-1850135

Dowdell, B. (n.d.). *How big pharma controls medicine.* Selfgrowth. https://www.selfgrowth.com/articles/how_big _pharma_controls_medicine

Dresden, D. (2020, January 1). *Top seven safe, effective natural antibiotics.* Medical News Today. https://www.medicalnewstoday.com/articles/3 21108

EcoWatch. (2016, September 20). *10 reasons to consider herbal medicine the next time you're not feeling well.* https://www.ecowatch.com/herbal-medicine-2009451657.html

Editors of Consumer Guide. (n.d.). *Alternative medicines for incontinence.* HowStuffWorks. https://health.howstuffworks.com/wellness/na tural-medicine/alternative/alternative-medicines-for-incontinence.htm

Egan, N. (n.d.). *Gas: Beat the bloat.* Bingham and Women's Hospital. https://www.brighamandwomens.org/patients-and-families/meals-and-nutrition/bwh-nutrition-and-wellness-hub/special-topics/gas-beat-the-bloat

8 simple, homemade herbal tea recipes. (n.d.). Simple Loose Leaf Tea Company. https://simplelooseleaf.com/blog/herbal-tea/herbal-tea-recipes/

Engels, J. (2014). *How medical school funding from big pharma impacts your health.* One Green Planet. https://www.onegreenplanet.org/natural-health/how-medical-school-funding-from-big-pharma-impacts-your-health/

Euro-American Connections & Homecare. (2017, January 10). *The benefits of transitioning to natural medicine: An interview with Dr. Ann Aresco, ND. Euro-American Connections & Homecare.* https://www.homecare4u.com/2017/01/transitioning-to-natural-medicine/

Fedyniak, L. G. (2007, February 1). *Medicine of the ancient Maya.* Vitality Magazine. https://vitalitymagazine.com/article/medicine-of-the-ancient-mayamedicine-ancient-maya/

5 astonishing herbs to promote testosterone level. (2020, February 19). Netmeds. https://www.netmeds.com/health-library/post/5-astonishing-herbs-to-promote-testosterone-level

5 herbs and spices for natural detoxification. (2020, December 9). Well Stated by Canyon Ranch. https://www.canyonranch.com/well-stated/post/5-herbs-and-spices-for-natural-detoxification/

Fletcher, J. (2018, March 17). *What is the best way to treat scabies at home?* Medical News Today.

https://www.medicalnewstoday.com/articles/3
21335#12-home-remedies-for-scabies

Fletcher, J. (2019, January 10). *What is an herbal tincture? Recipes and uses.* Medical News Today. https://www.medicalnewstoday.com/articles/3
24149

4 herbal remedies for postpartum anxiety. (2020, February 3). Dr. Emily Lesnak. https://www.dremilylesnak.com/new-blog/2020/1/10/4-herbal-remedies-for-postpartum-anxiety

Frotingham, S. (2018, July 12). *15 home remedies for allergies.* Healthline. https://www.healthline.com/health/home-remedies-for-allergies

Frothingham, S. (2019, May 24). *Which herbs help endometriosis symptoms?* Healthline. https://www.healthline.com/health/herbs-for-endometriosis

Frothingham, S. (2022, March 21). *Remove old scars: Top 10 medical remedies plus natural options.* Healthline. https://www.healthline.com/health/how-to-get-rid-of-old-scars

Galan, N. (2019, February 26). *8 herbs and supplements to help treat depression.* Medical News Today.

https://www.medicalnewstoday.com/articles/3
14421

Galloway, W. (2022, September 13). *Learn how to grow garlic in pots and you might never have to buy the store stuff again.* Apartment Therapy. https://www.apartmenttherapy.com/how-to-plant-garlic-in-contain-158494

Gateway Foundation. (2019, May 22). *Most commonly abused prescription drugs.* https://www.gatewayfoundation.org/addiction-blog/most-commonly-abused-prescription-drugs/

Gotter, A. (2019a, March 8). *Home remedies for ringworm.* Healthline. https://www.healthline.com/health/home-remedies-for-ringworm

Gotter, A. (2019b, October 25). *Home remedies for athlete's foot.* Healthline. https://www.healthline.com/health/home-remedies-for-athletes-foot

Gotter, A. (2023, March 24). *Home remedies for tonsillitis.* Healthline. https://www.healthline.com/health/home-remedies-for-tonsilitis

Greenman, D. E. (2018). *10 natural remedies for type 2 diabetes.* Stamford Health.

https://www.stamfordhealth.org/healthflash-blog/integrative-medicine/type-2-diabetes-natural-remedies/

Groves, M. N. (n.d.). *When and how to harvest herbs for medicinal use.* Storey Publishing. https://www.storey.com/article/harvest-herbs-medicinal-use/

Groza, D. (2022, November 15). *9 simple, natural ways to remove makeup.* Hello Glow. https://helloglow.co/9-simple-ways-to-remove-halloween-makeup/

Guide to medicinal plants found in the UK. (n.d.). Countryfile. https://www.countryfile.com/how-to/unusual-medicinal-plants-found-across-britain/

Harley, J. (2020, January 16). *10 best natural home remedies for IBS.* Mindset Health. https://www.mindsethealth.com/matter/10-best-natural-home-remedies-for-ibs

Harmon, W. (n.d.). *Homemade herbal tooth powder and toothpaste.* Traditional Cooking School by GNOWFGLINS. https://traditionalcookingschool.com/health-and-nutrition/homemade-herbal-tooth-powder-and-toothpaste/

Harris, N. (2022, December 5). *9 natural stretch mark treatments backed by science.* Parents. https://www.parents.com/pregnancy/my-body/best-natural-stretch-mark-treatments/

Hawkes, N. (2017, November 20). *Best herbal remedies to heal skin ulcers.* Nikki Hawkes. https://nikkihawkes.com/skin-ulcers-and-leg-ulcers/

Health | Natural remedies to help to live well with Addison's. (2017, September 30). Bognor Regis Post. https://www.bognorregispost.co.uk/2017/09/health-natural-remedies-help-live-well-addisons/

Health2Wellness. (2020). *Top 10 benefits of using herbal medicines.* https://www.health2wellnessblog.com/benefits-of-using-herbal-medicines/

Healthline Editorial Team. (2019, August 15). *Osteoporosis alternative treatments.* Healthline. https://www.healthline.com/health/osteoporosis-alternative-treatments

Healthline Editorial Team. (2021, January 29). *7 natural remedies for high cholesterol.* Healthline. https://www.healthline.com/health/heart-disease/natural-remedies-cholesterol

Herbal history: Roots of western herbalism. (n.d.). Herbal Academy. https://theherbalacademy.com/herbal-history/

Herbs that promote lymphatic drainage. (n.d.). Herbalism Roots. https://herbalismroots.com/herbs-promote-lymphatic-drainage/

Hill, A. (2023, February 14). *8 herbs and natural supplements for UTIs.* Healthline. https://www.healthline.com/nutrition/herbs-for-uti

Holland, K. (2017, February 7). *Alternative treatments for alzheimer's disease.* Healthline. https://www.healthline.com/health/alzheimers-disease/alternative-treatments

Home remedies for psoriasis relief. (2022, February 22). WebMD. https://www.webmd.com/skin-problems-and-treatments/psoriasis/ss/slideshow-home-remedies-for-psoriasis

How herbal medicine works. (n.d.). Dr. Schulze's. https://www.herbdoc.com/medicine-works

How to grow turmeric in pots | Turmeric plant care, uses and benefits. (n.d.). Balcony Garden Web. https://balconygardenweb.com/growing-turmeric-in-pots-how-to-grow-turmeric-care-uses-benefits

Huizen, J. (2023, January 12). *15 home remedies for acne.* Medical News Today. https://www.medicalnewstoday.com/articles/3 22455#home-remedies

Huizen, J. (2023, March 27). *12 home remedies for stomach pain.* Medical News Today. https://www.medicalnewstoday.com/articles/3 22047#Twenty-one-home-remedies

IARC Working Group on the Evaluation of Carcinogenic Risks to Humans. (2002). *Some traditional herbal medicines, some mycotoxins, naphthalene and styrene* (Vol. 82, pp. 43–64). IARC; Lyon, France. https://monographs.iarc.who.int/wp-content/uploads/2018/06/mono82-6a.pdf

Izuchukwu, O. J. (2018, February 28). *The history of African traditional medicine.* Academia. https://www.academia.edu/36040250/THE_H ISTORY_OF_AFRICAN_TRADITIONAL_ MEDICINE

Jeanroy, A. (2022a, March 9). *How to make a herbal tincture with vinegar, not alcohol.* The Spruce. https://www.thespruceeats.com/avoid-alcohol-and-make-vinegar-tinctures-1762274

Jeanroy, A. (2022b, April 1). *How to make herbal infusion.* The Spruce.

https://www.thespruceeats.com/how-to-make-an-herbal-infusion-1762142

Johnson, J. (2019, August 14). *Home remedies for relief from chickenpox symptoms.* Medical News Today. https://www.medicalnewstoday.com/articles/3 26051

K, A. (2020, July 27). *13 natural remedies for kidney infection that are available in your kitchen and garden.* Boldsky. https://www.boldsky.com/health/wellness/ho me-remedies-for-kidney-infection-134088.html

Kabala, J. (2020, December 14). *The 10 best herbs for liver health: Benefits and precautions.* Healthline. https://www.healthline.com/nutrition/herbs-for-liver

Kabir, S. (2016, April 10). *10 natural quick ways to get rid of cellulite.* Lifehack. https://www.lifehack.org/387147/10-natural-quick-ways-to-get-rid-of-cellulite

Kandola, A. (2018, February 10). *What are the best ways to get rid of nausea?* Medical News Today. https://www.medicalnewstoday.com/articles/3 20877

Kanthan, C. (2015, October 20). *How Rockefeller founded modern medicine and killed natural cures.* World Affairs. https://worldaffairs.blog/2015/10/20/how-rockefeller-founded-modern-medicine-and-killed-natural-cures/

Keeper of the Home. (2017, January 16). *The ultimate guide to homemade all-natural cleaning recipes.* https://keeperofthehome.org/homemade-all-natural-cleaning-recipes/

Kolen, R. (2017, July 13). *How to make herbal tinctures.* Mountain Rose Herbs. https://blog.mountainroseherbs.com/guide-tinctures-extracts

Krans, B. (2023, February 14). *Natural and home remedies for ulcers.* Healthline. https://www.healthline.com/health/natural-home-remedies-ulcers

Kubala, J. (2020, October 5). *The 10 best herbs to boost energy and focus.* Healthline. https://www.healthline.com/nutrition/herbs-for-energy

Kukreja, K. (2023, February 16). *Get rid of chapped lips fast using these 11 home remedies.* Stylecraze. https://www.stylecraze.com/articles/simple-homemade-tips-to-get-rid-of-chapped-lips/

Landau, M. D. (n.d.). *7 natural remedies for pain and pressure from sinus infections.* Everyday Health. https://www.everydayhealth.com/sinus-health-guide/natural-remedies-for-sinus-pain.aspx

Lee-Manes, C. (2022, April 3). *How to build a home apothecary: Using dried herbs, tinctures, & essential oils.* Homsted. https://www.homsted.com/blogs/homsted/how-to-build-a-home-apothecary-using-dried-herbs-t/

Leonard, J. (2017, May 31). *Which home remedy is best for bronchitis?* Medical News Today. https://www.medicalnewstoday.com/articles/317705

Lyle, W. (2014, May 16). *Herbal and holistic medicine in Latin America.* Western Kentucky University. https://digitalcommons.wku.edu/cgi/viewcontent.cgi?referer=&httpsredir=1&article=1482&context=stu_hon_theses

Macwelch, T. (2014, May 27). *Survival skills: 14 wild medicinal plants.* Outdoor Life. https://www.outdoorlife.com/blogs/survivalist/2014/05/survival-skills-14-wild-medicinal-plants/

Mann, F. (2019, May 10). *10 natural remedies for fungal skin infections.* A.Vogel. https://www.avogel.co.uk/health/skin/fungal-skin-infections/10-natural-remedies-for-fungal-skin-infections/

Maslowski, D. (n.d.). *DIY essential oils: Learn how to make your own essential oils.* DIY Natural. https://diynatural.com/diy-essential-oils/

May, B. (2017, June 13). *15 effective options for treating earache.* Medical News Today. https://www.medicalnewstoday.com/articles/3 12634

Mayo Clinic. (2022, October 15). *Prescription drug abuse.* https://www.mayoclinic.org/diseases-conditions/prescription-drug-abuse/symptoms-causes/syc-20376813

McBride, K. (2022, October 18). *The dangers of modern medicine.* Soapboxie. https://soapboxie.com/activism/The-dangers-of-modern-medicine

McCoy, K. (2017a, April 17). *Chlamydia symptoms + 5 natural treatments.* Dr. Axe. https://draxe.com/health/chlamydia-symptoms/

McCoy, K. (2017b, June 18). *What is hand, foot and mouth disease? +17 Natural treatments.* Dr. Axe. https://draxe.com/health/hand-foot-and-mouth-disease/

McDermott, A. (2017, August 16). *How to use carrier oils.* Healthline. https://www.healthline.com/health/carrier-oil

McDermott, A. (2018, June 15). *19 herbal remedies for hair growth.* Healthline. https://www.healthline.com/health/herbs-for-hair-growth

McDermott, A., & Collins, D. (2022, February 17). *Bee sting treatment: 6 home remedies.* Healthline. https://www.healthline.com/health/outdoor-health/home-remedies-for-bee-stings

McDermott, A., & Santos-Longhurt, A. (2023, January 20). *11 home remedies for vaginal yeast infections.* Healthline. https://www.healthline.com/health/womens-health/yeast-infection-home-remedy

Metcalf, E. (n.d.). *Natural remedies for dandruff.* WebMD. https://www.webmd.com/skin-problems-and-treatments/features/natural-fixes

Mikulic, M. (2023, January 3). *Revenues of top 10 national pharmaceutical markets worldwide in 2021.* Statista. https://www.statista.com/statistics/266469/revenues-of-the-top-10-global-pharmaceutical-markets/

Mortlock, S. (2019, January 30). *Health and herbs in the dark ages.* The Biomedical Scientist Magazine of the IBMS. https://thebiomedicalscientist.net/science/health-and-herbs-dark-ages

Mother Earth Living Staff. (2022, January 15). *4 bulk herb wholesalers you can trust*. Mother Earth Living. https://www.motherearthliving.com/health-and-wellness/bulk-herb-wholesalers-you-can-trust-zmez16jazolc

Mousa, H. A.-L. (2016). Prevention and treatment of influenza, influenza-like illness, and common cold by herbal, complementary, and natural therapies. *Journal of Evidence-Based Complementary & Alternative Medicine, 22*(1), 166–174. https://doi.org/10.1177/2156587216641831

Murphy, S. (2020, May 7). *13 natural remedies for severe asthma*. Healthline. https://www.healthline.com/health/severe-asthma/natural-remedies

The National Gardening Association. (n.d.). *The 2012 USDA hardiness zone map* [Map]. https://garden.org/nga/zipzone/2012/

Naser, S. (2023, March 6). *10 home remedies to get rid of ganglion cysts + causes and medical treatment*. Stylecraze. https://www.stylecraze.com/articles/ganglion-cyst-treatment/

Natural cough remedies. (n.d.). WebMD. https://www.webmd.com/cold-and-flu/ss/slideshow-natural-cough-remedies

Natural remedies to fight cavities. (2019, September 3). Steven K. Okamoto. https://www.okamotodds.com/blog/2019/9/3/natural-remedies-to-fight-cavities/

Naturopath. (2017, April 23). *Natural therapies for motor neuron disease.* SuperPharmacy. https://www.superpharmacy.com.au/blog/natural-therapies-for-motor-neuron-disease

Nayyar, N. (n.d.). *Herbal medicine: How does it work?* Womenfitness. https://www.womenfitness.net/herbalmed.htm

Neil's Yard Remedies. (2019, November 12). *Natural treatments for post-traumatic stress disorder.* Mother Earth Living. https://www.motherearthliving.com/health-and-wellness/natural-remedies/PTSD-ze0z1901zcoy/

New Delhi Television. (2018, August 20). *6 home remedies for gas that are sure to give relief.* https://food.ndtv.com/health/6-home-remedies-for-gas-that-are-sure-to-give-relief-1643392

Nunez, K. (2022, February 22). *16 natural home remedies for warts.* Healthline. https://www.healthline.com/health/home-remedies-for-warts

Oberg, B. (2012, May 8). *Three herbs everyone with BPD should know about.* HealthyPlace. https://www.healthyplace.com/blogs/borderlin e/2012/05/three-herbs-everyone-with-bpd-should-know-about

Panchal, B. (2023, February 20). *9 home remedies for cold sores.* Holland & Barrett. https://www.hollandandbarrett.com/the-health-hub/natural-beauty/skincare/lip-care/9-home-remedies-for-cold-sores/

Parpia, R. (2018, April 15). *Big pharma pays universities for most medical research in U.S. today.* The Vaccine Reaction. https://thevaccinereaction.org/2018/04/big-pharma-pays-universities-for-most-medical-research-in-u-s-today/

Pastorek, G. (n.d.). *5 natural remedies for poison ivy rashes.* Allegheny-Kiski Health Foundation. https://akhealth.org/natural-remedies-for-poison-ivy/

Patiry, M. (n.d.). *Homemade herbal antibiotic—No prescription necessary!* PaleoHacks. https://blog.paleohacks.com/homemade-herbal-antibiotic/

Petre, A., & Ajmera, R. (2023, March 29). *10 natural sleep aids for better sleep in 2023.* Healthline.

https://www.healthline.com/nutrition/sleep-aids#passionflower

Petre, A, & Link, R. (2022, June 21). *9 natural sleep aids that may help you get some shut-eye in 2022.* Healthline. https://www.healthline.com/nutrition/sleep-aids

Petrovska, B. B. (2012). Historical review of medicinal plants' usage. *Pharmacognosy Reviews, 6*(11), 1. https://doi.org/10.4103/0973-7847.95849

Ponsford, S. (2017, December 14). *How to treat a toothache at home.* Medical News Today. https://www.medicalnewstoday.com/articles/320315

Potter, D., & Brind'Amour, K. (2020, July 7). *Going herbal: Vitamins and supplements for multiple sclerosis.* Healthline. https://www.healthline.com/health/multiple-sclerosis/going-herbal-vitamins-and-supplements-for-multiple-sclerosis

Power of Positivity. (2022, May 7). *How to grow herbs at home: An easy 7 step guide.* https://www.powerofpositivity.com/how-to-grow-herbs-at-home/

Pristyn Care Team. (2023, February 18). *10 remedies that can cure hiatal hernia naturally.* Pristyn Care.

https://www.pristyncare.com/blog/natural-remedies-to-cure-hiatal-hernia-pc0135/

Purple Herbal. (2011, June 11). *10 easy to find wild medicinal herbs*. https://purpleherbal.wordpress.com/2011/06/11/10-easy-to-find-wild-medicinal-herbs/

Rafatjah, S. (2019, October 23). *How to cure hypothyroidism permanently*. PrimeHealth. https://primehealthdenver.com/how-to-cure-hypothyroidism-permanently/

Rajesh, L. (2023, February 2). *19 ways to remove dark circles*. Femina. https://www.femina.in/beauty/skin/remove-dark-circles-57696.html

Rana, S. (2018a, April 20). *How to remove kidney stones naturally? 8 ways to cleanse your kidneys*. New Delhi Television. https://food.ndtv.com/food-drinks/how-to-remove-kidney-stones-naturally-8-ways-to-cleanse-your-kidneys-1693610

Rana, S. (2018b, April 26). *9 effective home remedies to stop nose bleeding*. New Delhi Television. https://food.ndtv.com/health/effective-home-remedies-to-stop-nose-bleeding-1842722

Reis, M. (2022, February). *6 natural remedies to get rid of gallstones*. Tua Saúde.

https://www.tuasaude.com/en/natural-
remedies-for-gallstones/

Richards, L. (2023, January 20). *9 herbs for anxiety.*
Medical   News   Today.
https://www.medicalnewstoday.com/articles/h
erbs-for-anxiety

Robbins, K. (2014, September 10). *Herbal medicine:
History of Chinese herbal medicine.* DailyU.
http://www.dailyu.com/health/herbal-
medicine-history-of-chinese-herbal-medicine/

Roberts-Grey, G. (2017, November 15). *5 natural
remedies for rosacea.* Everyday Health.
https://www.everydayhealth.com/skin-
beauty/rosacea/5-natural-remedies-rosacea/

Sacasas, C. (2019, February 22). *10 must-have herbs to start
your own home apothecary for natural wellness.* Lone
Star   Botanicals.
https://www.lonestarbotanicals.com/home-
apothecary/

Sawyers, T. (2019, March 7). *Top 5 best male yeast infection
home   remedies.*   Healthline.
https://www.healthline.com/health/male-
yeast-infection-home-remedy

Sellami, M., Slimeni, O., Pokrywka, A., Kuvačić, G.,
Hayes, L. D., Milic, M., & Padulo, J. (2022).
Herbal medicine for sports: A review. *Journal of*

the *International Society of Sports Nutrition, 15*(15), 14. https://doi.org/10.1186/s12970-018-0218-y

7 superb home remedies to get rid of mouth ulcers. (2018, August 24). NDTV Food. https://food.ndtv.com/food-drinks/7-superb-home-remedies-to-get-rid-of-mouth-ulcers-1443372

SF Gate Contributor. (2020, June 19). *How to grow cayenne peppers in a container.* SF Gate. https://homeguides.sfgate.com/grow-cayenne-peppers-container-47525.html

Shetty, P. (2010, May 27). *Integrating modern and traditional medicine: Facts and figures.* SciDev.Net. https://www.scidev.net/global/features/integrating-modern-and-traditional-medicine-facts-and-figures/

Shrotri, S. (n.d.). *6-ingredient all natural aloe vera face cream.* Vegan First. https://www.veganfirst.com/recipe/diy-beauty-pamper-yourself-with-a-homemade-face-cream-

SingleCare Team. (2022, October 12). *24 home remedies for constipation.* The Checkup. https://www.singlecare.com/blog/home-remedies-for-constipation/

SingleCare Team. (2022, December 5). *15 home remedies for toenail fungus*. The Checkup. https://www.singlecare.com/blog/home-remedies-for-toenail-fungus/

Sinha, R. (2023, February 1). *10 simple homemade body wash recipes*. Stylecraze. https://www.stylecraze.com/articles/simple-homemade-body-wash-recipes/

Snyder, C. (2021, June 23). *5 impressive herbs that help balance your hormones*. Healthline. https://www.healthline.com/nutrition/herbs-that-balance-hormones

Staughton, J. (2020, January 29). *15 best herbal teas and their health benefits*. Organic Facts. https://www.organicfacts.net/health-benefits/herbs-and-spices/types-of-herbal-tea.html

Stickler, T. (2020, June 4). *Migraine herbal home remedies from around the world*. Healthline. https://www.healthline.com/health/migraine-herbal-home-remedies-from-around-the-world

Stone, K. (2019, May 8). *How to make your own effective herbal remedies*. Stone Family Farmstead. https://www.stonefamilyfarmstead.com/how-to-make-your-own-effective-herbal-remedies/

Sturluson, T. (2014, January 30). *History of herbal medicine.* The Herbal Resource. https://www.herbal-supplement-resource.com/history-of-herbal-medicine/

Sutton, J. (2019, August 29). *30 foods and herbs that may boost female sex drive.* Healthline. https://www.healthline.com/health/sex-drive-foods-female

Sziraczki, A. (n.d.). *Natural remedies for scarlet fever.* Raising Toxin Free Children. https://www.raisingtoxinfreechildren.com/natural-remedies-for-scarlet-fever/

Taggar, M. (2022, March 11). *10 ways to help prevent wrinkles.* Holland & Barrett. https://www.hollandandbarrett.com/the-health-hub/natural-beauty/skincare/anti-ageing/six-healthy-habits-help-ward-off-wrinkles/

10 home remedies for gum disease. (n.d.). Guardian Direct. https://www.guardiandirect.com/dental-care/10-home-remedies-gum-disease

Teta, J. S., & Bessinger, J. (2014, September 19). *Natural remedies for celiac disease.* Mother Earth Living. https://www.motherearthliving.com/health-and-wellness/natural-remedies/natural-remedies-for-celiac-disease-ze0z1409zdeb/

22 most dangerous FDA approved drugs. (2017, October 17). Cinnamon Vogue Inc. https://cinnamonvogue.com/blog/22-most-dangerous-fda-approved-drugs/

Villegas, H. (2018). *How to forage edible and wild plants successfully and safely: 15 tips for wild harvesting.* Healing Harvest Homestead. https://healingharvesthomestead.com/home/2018/4/14/tips-for-wild-harvesting-medicinal-herbs-how-to-forage-herbs-successfully-and-safely

Visser, M. (2013, January 9). *How to make your own herbal antibiotics at home.* Growing up Herbal. https://growingupherbal.com/how-to-make-your-own-herbal-antibiotics-at-home/

Visser, M. (2018, August 27). *What every herbalist should know about herbal preparation shelf life.* Herbal Academy. https://theherbalacademy.com/herbal-preparation-shelf-life/

Watson, K. (2019, March 8). *10 home remedies for vertigo.* Healthline. https://www.healthline.com/health/home-remedies-for-vertigo

Watson, K. (2023, February 16). *32 home remedies for herpes simplex virus 1 and virus 2.* Healthline.

https://www.healthline.com/health/sexually-transmitted-diseases/home-remedies-for-herpes

Webber, J. (n.d.). *9 hero herbs to help naturally cure your hangover.* Pukka Herbs. https://www.pukkaherbs.com/us/en/wellbeing-articles/9-hero-herbs-to-help-naturally-cure-your-hangover

WebMD Editorial Contributors. (n.d.). *12 natural treatment tips for colds and flu.* WebMD. https://www.webmd.com/cold-and-flu/12-tips-prevent-colds-flu-1

WebMD Editorial Contributors. (n.d.). *Alternative treatments for insomnia.* WebMD. https://www.webmd.com/sleep-disorders/alternative-treatments-for-insomnia

Weil, A. (2011, May 25). *Why plants are (usually) better than drugs.* HuffPost. https://www.huffpost.com/entry/why-plants-are-usually-be_b_785139

Weiser-Alexander, K. (2021, December). *Native American medicine.* Legends of America. https://www.legendsofamerica.com/na-medicine/

Welz, A. N., Emberger-Klein, A., & Menrad, K. (2018). Why people use herbal medicine: Insights from a focus-group study in Germany. *BMC*

Complementary and Alternative Medicine, *18*(1). https://doi.org/10.1186/s12906-018-2160-6

Westover, J. (n.d.). *Growing purple coneflowers in containers.* SF Gate. https://homeguides.sfgate.com/growing-purple-coneflowers-containers-60904.html

What is Ayurveda? The history of Ayurveda. (n.d.). Ayurvedic India. https://www.ayurvedicindia.info/history-of-ayurveda/

White, A. (2019, March 7). *How to treat dry mouth at home.* Healthline. https://www.healthline.com/health/dry-mouth-remedies

Wigglesworth, S. (2020, December 30). *How to grow ginger indoors.* Yankee Magazine. https://newengland.com/today/living/gardening/how-to-grow-ginger-indoors/

Wong, C. (2022a, June 28). *Herbs and supplements for fibromyalgia.* Verywell Health. https://www.verywellhealth.com/herbs-and-supplements-for-fibromyalgia-88228

Wong, C. (2022b, November 18). *Natural burn remedies and ointments.* Verywell Health. https://www.verywellhealth.com/burn-remedies-89945

Wood, M. (n.d.). *How to make a tincture (+alcohol-free option!).* Our Inspired Roots. https://ourinspiredroots.com/how-to-make-a-tincture/

Woyka, J. (2020, September). *Complementary & alternative therapies: Non hormonal prescribed treatments.* Women's Health Concern. https://www.womens-health-concern.org/wp-content/uploads/2022/12/03-WHC-FACTSHEET-Complementary-And-Alternative-Therapies-NOV2022-B.pdf

Zapf, M., & Phoenix, K. (2020, August 27). *Natural remedies to get rid of head lice.* Good Housekeeping. https://www.goodhousekeeping.com/health/a20707336/natural-head-lice-remedy/

Image References

Canty, J. (2020, November 28). [*Woman in pink panty and bra*] [Image]. Unsplash. https://unsplash.com/photos/dF8jzk6GdQc

Danilina, A. (2018, July 20). *Her wonderland* [Image]. Unsplash. https://unsplash.com/photos/zgohOdeKpnA

Drndarski, T. (2020, January 22). *Fresh garlic on dark background* [Image]. Unsplash. https://unsplash.com/photos/2yNBQFwZCA 8

Eduardo Cano Photo Co. (2019, November 12). *Herbal tea mint drink* [Image]. Unsplash. https://unsplash.com/photos/KkvLtNL61co

Etactics Inc. (2022, July 28). [*A miniature figure with a syringe and vial*] [Image]. Unsplash. https://unsplash.com/photos/5izv95wuK3g

Green, V. (2020, September 11). [*Yellow flower with green leaves*] [Image]. Unsplash. https://unsplash.com/photos/i-uBAOo_BBA

Grianghraf. (2021, September 28). [*Purple, yellow, and white flower*] [Image]. Unsplash. https://unsplash.com/photos/MVQqPxRS5xk

Haupt, M. (2020, March 27). *A yellow flower that looks like fireworks* [Image]. Unsplash. https://unsplash.com/photos/xMH927YJyq4

Kim, B. (2018, December 26). [*Assorted-item lot*] [Image]. Unsplash. https://unsplash.com/photos/ur2zmbseUIA

Kolleshi, A. (2018, May 29). *Dentist student* [Image]. Unsplash. https://unsplash.com/photos/7jjnJ-QA9fY

Martinez, J. (2019, May 21). [*Selective focus photography of a cactus*] [Image]. Unsplash. https://unsplash.com/photos/ziNvM5dVDaU

Milde-Jachowska, P. (2021, November 12). *Amber glass* [Image]. Unsplash. https://unsplash.com/photos/WaVHS5UKfm E

Olofsson, E. (2020, September 22). [*Person holding brown glass bottle*] [Image]. Unsplash. https://unsplash.com/photos/HvC6jKUtWgU

Petric, M. (2017, February 24). *Making rosehip tea* [Image]. Unsplash. https://unsplash.com/photos/A4dhzVLC_Do

Romanovski, F. (2021, May 10). *Selfmade sorrel pesto. Enjoy* [Image]. Unsplash. https://unsplash.com/photos/Qbu9QesmTIQ

Rinaldi, M. (2019, January 18). [*Clear glass mug on tray*] [Image]. Unsplash. https://unsplash.com/photos/FmgZ5xzDG-s

Seymour, M. (2020, June 26). [*Purple flower in tilt shift lens*] [Image]. Unsplash. https://unsplash.com/photos/u5r8wtEmI80

Spiske, M. (2018, April 10). [*Green leafed seedlings in black plastic pots*] [Image]. Unsplash. https://unsplash.com/photos/4PG6wLlVag4

Stupnytska, Y. (2021, June 18). [*White and yellow flowers in tilt-shift lens*] [Image]. Unsplash. https://unsplash.com/photos/0f3AfGPzgpY

Topp, J. (2021, June 12). [*Brown and white food on white ceramic plate*] [Image]. Unsplash. https://unsplash.com/photos/Xz4M49O8QcE

Printed in Great Britain
by Amazon

34069935R00165